Increase your

Learn how to have
Learn how to ha

A book for women of all ages

by Sandra Cabot MD

Copyright © 2012 Dr. Sandra Cabot
Published by SCB Inc. - United States of America

www.sandracabot.com
www.liverdoctor.com

ISBN 978-0-9829336-9-5

SELF-HELP / Sexual Instruction
HEALTH & FITNESS / Women's Health
HEALTH & FITNESS / Sexuality

Love, Libido , Sex Drive, Sex Therapy, Orgasm, Vaginal Problems, Painful Sex

Disclaimer

The suggestions, ideas and treatments described in this book must not replace the care and direct supervision of a trained healthcare professional. All problems and concerns regarding your health require medical supervision by a medical doctor. If you have any pre-existing medical disorders, you must consult your own doctor before following the suggestions in this book. If you are taking any prescribed medications, you should check with your own doctor before using the recommendations in this book.

Notice of Rights

Contents

Introduction

I decided to write a book on love and sex because, over more than 30 years of practising medicine, I have often been asked for help to overcome sexual problems by many of my female patients.

I see a lot of women with hormonal problems ranging from menopause and polycystic ovarian syndrome to unexplained infertility and weight problems. During the history taking, many women often complain that they have lost their interest in sex and they are not happy about this.

I am not a sex therapist but I do have an enormous amount of clinical experience in helping women with hormonal problems. If your sex hormones are out of balance, your sex life will suffer and this book explains how to use bio-identical hormones to restore a normal and healthy balance of sex hormones; it also explains how you can maximize the health of your sexual organs using nutritional medicine. If you are in poor health or you *feel old*, your sex life will suffer, as this will impact adversely upon your hormones and your mental and emotional health.

I have found that self esteem has a huge influence on a woman's sexual identity and I have included a few case histories to illustrate this point. I do hope this book helps you to improve your self esteem and inspires you to be the best you can be in the bedroom and in your daily life. Education about your body and its sexual parts is fundamental to improving your sex life.

I also wrote this book because of the ageing population of women who have to face greater challenges to be able to stay young, healthy and sexy. It is mind boggling to think that at the beginning of the 20th century (that's only 110 years ago), the average life span of a woman was less than 50 years. Today in the year 2011, the average life span of a woman has increased to 80 years; so merely just over 100 years ago a woman of 50 was considered old and hardly a sexual creature. Today a woman of 50 is considered middle aged with the potential to enjoy a fulfilling sexual relationship. She will need to be healthy and, as she ages, she will usually need help with her hormones which have declined to very low levels.

My own mother is 84 years of age and she is no longer interested in sex or the opposite sex, apart from friendship. She is still a formidable woman who has a sharp mind and an abundant and wise personality. She has had three husbands, and as they have all passed away, she vindicates the statistics that women outlive men!

When I look at my mother I am inspired because, thanks to nutritional supplements and a good diet, she is healthy, and just as importantly, she has accepted herself for the incredible human being that she is; in other words she has good self esteem.

We are both fiery and strong women and we sometimes clash and have a disagreement. I think she is still the only person who can break my heart, as if we do have a spat, the day after I will give her flowers and money, which I put in the trophy cup I gave her which is inscribed with the words *The Best Mother in the World.*

My mother has arrived at the age where she lives for her three daughters and money has become sexier than sex!

> *I dedicate this book to my mother Jacqueline,*
> *she will always be my inspiration.*

1. Mars and Venus or XY and XX ?

When it comes to heterosexual sex and love I think that generally speaking, men and women are different. In same sex couples there is usually the more male character and the more female character both in life behavior and in the bedroom. But same sex couples can reverse roles so maybe they can have more fun and variety than heterosexual couples.

There have been thousands of books written on the fundamental differences between the sexes, the most famous being *Men are from Mars and Women are from Venus* written by John Gray. This book has sold over 7 million copies, which is a testimonial to just how difficult it can be for the two sexes to see things in the same context. Sometimes it can become very cerebral and complicated and this can become a little dreary. When it all gets too hard, remember the little frog who says "Don't try to understand me, just love me!" I agree, love is more powerful than our thoughts and can heal all wounds.

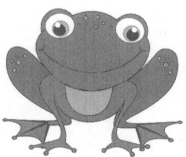

Don't try to understand me,
just love me!

I am not an astrologer but I do remember my mother telling me that Mars is the planet of fire and war and Venus is the planet of love and beauty – makes sense then, as far as Gray's book title goes.

Women tend to be more mental (or in their brain) about sex, whereas men tend to think and feel sex below the waist; in other words men are more animal and their basic sexual instinct is more physically centered around their genital organs. During a session of love making women are often thinking about something whilst a man is totally focused on the physical sensation. Here is a little scene to illustrate this extremely common pattern of behavior.

One Monday morning a married couple is getting ready for work and while the husband is having a shower upstairs the wife is in the kitchen cooking the breakfast. The husband comes down the stairs fully dressed and looking smart and professional. His wife is still in her bath robe trying to catch up with the demands of the day. As soon as she sees her husband she says to him "Quick we must have sex immediately!" He is very happy about this and quickly undresses himself and pulls off her robe, lays her on the kitchen table and starts to have sex – the ever ready male! So they have good sex and once it is all over, he relaxes and says to his wife, "Darling that was wonderful and fabulous, why were you so spontaneous?" She replies very dryly and casually "Oh the egg timer is broken!" Yes, while he was getting his rocks off, she was all the time in her mind thinking about getting the eggs correctly cooked and then getting dressed in time for work!

I have found that it is often true that women are in their thoughts during sex when they really need to stop thinking and instead be focusing on their body and its sensual parts.

Over the nearly 40 years that I have been a medical doctor I have observed some interesting differences between the sexes –

- None of my male patients have ever asked me for help to improve their libido (sexual drive); instead they ask for help to improve their sexual performance.

- None of my female patients have ever asked for help to improve their sexual performance; instead they ask for help to improve their libido and/or their ability to achieve orgasms and sexual satisfaction.

- Men ask for help with their sexual performance primarily for their own ego and satisfaction and then, that of their partner.
- Women often respond to my explanation that *this treatment will help your libido* with the statement "Oh my husband will be pleased!" I find this curious, as I have never heard a man say that.
- Women tend to lack or lose interest in sex far more than men do – do we blame it on the planets or on our hormonal differences or is it due to our different sex chromosomes; I tend to think it's the latter, as, after all, our DNA is the genetic code that makes us who we are.

When it comes to our sex chromosomes, women have two X chromosomes (XX), men have only one X and the other male sex chromosome is a Y (thus a male's sex chromosomes are XY). It is fascinating to compare the X and the Y chromosomes as they are very different. The Y chromosome is much smaller in size than the X chromosome and has only 70 to 200 genes on it (we are still mapping the finer details of the human genome).

The X chromosome has around 2000 genes on it so that means it has 15 times as many genes on it than the Y chromosome. Now girls, this gives us something to brag about!

Sex Chromosomes

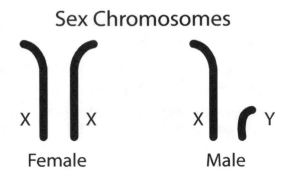

X   X   X   Y
Female   Male

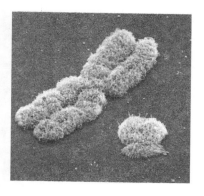

Picture of male and female sex chromosomes -
X chromosome on the left and Y chromosome on the right.

Doesn't the Y chromosome look cute?

Genetic researchers have worked out that the genome (entire structure of chromosomes and genes) in men and women is different by about 1 to 2 percent. This may not sound like a large amount of difference. But when you think about the fact that the differences between the genome of the human male and the male chimpanzee is also 1 to 2 percent, you have got to wonder!

Chromosome Variance

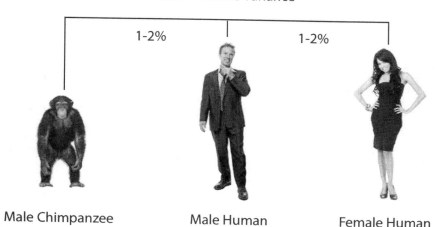

1-2%   1-2%

Male Chimpanzee   Male Human   Female Human

Honey, I feel confused, maybe we should go to a good sex therapist after all?

I sometimes jokingly ask the question "Y are men different to women?" The answer is "Because men have the Y chromosome – that's Y they are different". It may sound corny or clichéd, but it is a genetic difference that could play out in the bedroom!

Maybe the Y chromosome lacks some of the *feeling soft* genes that exist on X chromosomes. Of course I am generalizing but it is fun!

I once told a guy "Hey, you should see the Y chromosome, it's so small and it looks kind of cute and fragile". I was surprised and somewhat perplexed by his response, which was "Well now I know why size does not matter and it's not my fault!"

Let's not be too serious, as we aim to bring the male and female sex together in perfect sexual balance and enjoyment.

I'm NOT in the mood!

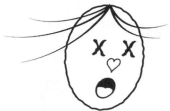
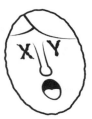

What's MOOD got to do with it?

2. Understanding your erogenous zones

A woman's sexual organs are called the genitalia, meaning the genital organs. They consist of the vagina and the vulva. The vagina is an internal tube shaped cavity connecting the outside to the cervix of the uterus. The cervix is the opening to the uterus. The vagina is separate from the vulva.

The vulva is outside the body and includes all the outer genitals you can see when you open your legs and look in the mirror. The appearance of the vulva can vary quite a lot between different women and all these variations are considered normal. It can be compared to other anatomical variations such as some women have big hips, some have small hips, some have a large nose, some have a small nose, some have large pendulous breasts, some have perky compact breasts and some have very little breast tissue.

The Vulva

The word vulva means *covering*, which is appropriate as it covers and protects the opening of the vagina and the opening to the bladder. The opening to the bladder's exit tube is called the urethral meatus and this is where urine exits.

The vulva consists of the following parts:

• The outer lips (the labia majora). The skin of the outer lips contains hair follicles and glands that secrete sweat and a waxy liquid called sebum

• The inner lips (the labia minora). These are smaller and thinner than the outer lips and are hairless. The appearance and size of the inner lips can vary greatly between normal women

• The edges of both lips contain tiny glands that secrete oily fluid essential to the health of the lips. These glands can appear as very tiny white lumps, which is normal

• The vestibule – this is the area that exists between the inner lips

In the middle of the vestibule we find the openings of the vagina and urinary tract. The vestibule has an extremely rich blood and nerve supply and, during sexual arousal, the vestibule and inner lips become engorged with blood.

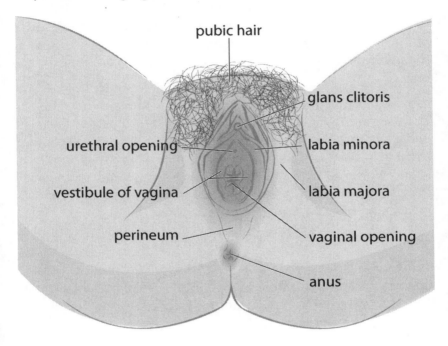

- The clitoris is generally viewed by women as a small raised firm nub of tissue at the top of the inner lips. It looks small right? Yes it does and you may think you have been short changed compared to men, but in reality the clitoris is much larger than the ¼ inch tip you can see and feel. This nub of tissue is called the glans clitoris.

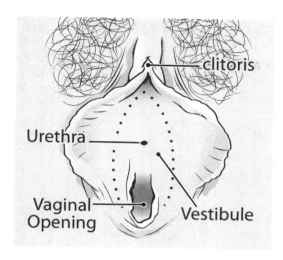

The glans clitoris is attached to a shaft around 1 inch long that connects to your pubic bone and this shaft divides into 2 roots known as crura that attach to the pelvic bones. You cannot see the shaft and the roots as they are covered by tissue. The clitoris is supplied by thousands of nerve endings which make it extremely sensitive to touch. Some women find that direct stimulation of the glans clitoris is too strong and almost painful and they find that it feels much better if their partner gently stimulates the shaft of the clitoris. If your clitoris is extremely sensitive, ask your partner to be very gentle and only touch you lightly, especially to begin with.

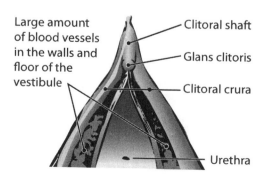

The Clitoris - approximatley 8,000 nerve endings meet here

Many women can achieve orgasm from stimulation of the clitoris either by their partner or by their own fingers or a vibrator. This is a good thing, as more than half of all women fail to achieve orgasm from vaginal intercourse. Guess what? Men do not know this and maybe it is hard for them to take!

During sexual arousal the clitoris swells to around double its size because it has such a huge blood supply. Thus a healthy blood circulation is essential to a good sexual response. Blood can flow into and out of the clitoris causing it to vary in size and this enables some women to have multiple orgasms.

Things that reduce the blood supply such as diabetes, high blood pressure or smoking can reduce your ability to have clitoral orgasms. Testosterone therapy can increase the size and sensitivity of the clitoris and women with very low testosterone levels may have problems achieving orgasm.

The G Spot

The G spot is famous but also controversial, as there is still a lot of discussion as to where it is and if it really exists. I have been told by couples that it's a lot of fun trying to find the G spot!

This famous spot is thought to be the most sexually sensitive and the most arousing spot for some women, but not for all women.

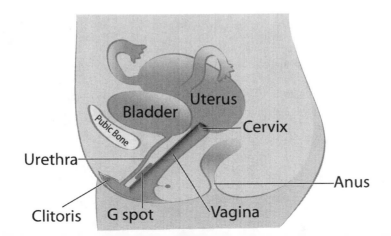

So where is the G spot thought to be located?

It is thought to be an area of tissue in the lower front wall of the vagina just near the urethra. This area is smooth and not wrinkly like the rest of the vagina. Some researchers think that the G spot is the underneath part of the clitoris when it is stimulated or pressured through the front wall of the vagina.

The G spot could also be partly found in the tissue just underneath the skin of the vestibule – this is called the bulb of the vestibule. This tissue has an extremely rich blood supply and when blood flows into this tissue the vestibule enlarges and stiffens, you could say like a form of female erection. The G spot is only obvious if you are sexually aroused, so don't go on a finding expedition if you are not! You can search for the G spot by rubbing along the lower front wall inside your vagina with two fingers, a dildo or vibrator. Remember it's not high up in the vagina near the cervix.

Some women report experiencing wonderful sensations from the G spot if they have rear entry vaginal sex or if they are on top of their partner.

Some women have never found their G spot but still enjoy a great sex life with plenty of orgasms, so do not worry if you cannot find it – we are all different and that is normal.

Orgasms

You may be surprised, and possibly relieved, to know that more than half of all women do not orgasm with vaginal intercourse. This means that if sex is restricted to only the insertion of the penis into the vagina and thrusting of the penis inside the vagina, the majority of women will not experience an orgasm – in other words they will not climax. Was God a male chauvinist? I don't think so, it's just that there are many different ways to have an orgasm and women are different in the way they achieve the elusive orgasm. It's just plain normal to be different!

The normal differences are-

- Some women have much more difficulty achieving orgasms than others and we don't always know why
- Women achieve orgasm by different mechanisms
- Some women have multiple orgasms routinely whilst others never have more than one during a sexual encounter
- The intensity of orgasms can vary a lot in one woman at different times and between different women. It may be a little whimper or it may be an intense pleasurable volcano.

Although it feels good to have an orgasm, especially an intense one that releases tension, it is not essential to have an orgasm every time you have sex; indeed it is not the norm for most women. You can be sexually fulfilled even if you do not have an orgasm. There are no rules to follow and no stereotype you should try to emulate.

What physical changes happen in your body during an orgasm?

The founders of modern day sexual medicine, Masters and Johnson, first described the four stages of sexual response in women in 1966. These stages gave us a general physiological picture; however remember that every woman is different, so if you do not fit into these stages exactly, don't worry, you are still normal. The most important thing about sex is to enjoy it; it's meant to be fun and relaxing! If you try too hard to be a *femme fatale* or to have multiple orgasms, you will miss out, as you will be too much in your head and not enough in your pelvis.

The first stage – excitement

During stage one you become aroused and this causes the vulva to swell with blood – this is called engorgement. A natural chemical called Nitric Oxide (NO) is produced in the walls of the blood vessels supplying the vulva in increased amounts. NO is a potent dilator of blood vessels and when the arteries open up wider, the circulation of blood increases dramatically and the vulva swells. This whole area feels full, warm and much more responsive. Fluid then starts to be secreted from the lining of the vagina and vulva to produce the much needed lubrication. The amount of fluid secreted can vary a lot and that is why lubricants are sometimes required.

The upper part of the vagina expands from its normally collapsed state to a cavity wide enough to accommodate an erect penis. The uterus and cervix rise up in the pelvic cavity to make room for the erect penis. The body produces extra adrenalin, which causes the pulse rate to increase, the blood pressure to rise, the muscles become poised and mental excitement is heightened. This is the best time for your partner to stimulate your clitoris – you are now ready to respond. You may need to teach your partner to wait until you are at this point before your clitoris is touched, as if it's done too early or too roughly it will not feel right and indeed may be unpleasant.

We need to teach men about foreplay, as for most men it's not instinctual; they have either read about it in a magazine or talked to their mates or experimented on other women who were non-communicative. Your partner will probably be relieved to get instructive tips from you. You may have heard the joke – A woman asks a man "How long does it take for a woman to orgasm?" The man replies "Who cares!" Thankfully most men are not like that, however there are some cultures where only men's desires and satisfaction are considered important.

Many women experiment with a vibrator at some stage in their life and the advantages include –

* Learning about your own body and it's responses
* The ability to be able to do something about your own arousal when you want to
* Spare batteries are cheap and uncomplicated
* They have an on and off switch you can control
* They don't fall asleep at the end of stage one

17

The second stage - plateau

When the first stage is complete and the vulva is engorged with blood, the excitement starts to level off. The tissues around the lower vagina swell thus narrowing the vagina and squeeze the penis and this feels good to both partners. During the plateau phase the uterus is pushed up further and the upper part of the vagina expands more so that the penis is able to thrust in deeper. The labia minora (inner lips) expand and swell changing color to a deeper red. The plateau phase varies in duration and a woman may go back into the excitement phase for a while and then back into the plateau phase.

The third stage – orgasm

When orgasm occurs there is intense pleasure accompanied by contractions of the muscles around the vagina and in the tissues between the vagina and anus. For many women, orgasm cannot be produced by vaginal intercourse alone and their partner needs to stimulate the clitoris at the same time. Some women can have an orgasm from vaginal stimulation alone, especially from stimulation of an area in the front part of the lower vagina – this is thought to be the elusive G spot.

There are no hard and fast or black and white rules – we are all different. It is normal for some women to experience a big variation in their orgasms. Some orgasms may be a very short lived fleeting pleasure whilst other orgasms may be sustained and intense and even result in multiple orgasms.

The fourth stage – resolution

This is the final stage of the sexual response and lasts 10 to 15 seconds only. During this phase all the sexual organs return back to their normal shape and size. The vaginal walls thin, the vaginal cavity collapses, the labia return back to normal size and color and the clitoris shrinks back to its normal size. The resolution phase is due to the draining of the excess blood away from the genital area.

Hormonal changes during orgasm

What happens to hormone levels during an orgasm is astounding – when you climax, your brain and your body is flooded with the hormones dopamine and oxytocin. Dopamine is the chemical that makes us feel stimulated, focused and rewarded so that satisfaction is guaranteed. The natural high from an orgasm can be really intense due to these high dopamine levels and you feel fulfilled. Studies have shown that the brain scans of people experiencing an intense orgasm look like the scans of people having a high from some drugs – but this time it's a natural high free of dangerous side effects. The chemistry of sex happens more in our brain (between our ears) than it does between our legs.

During an orgasm the amount of activity in the outer layer of the brain (the cortex) decreases and the amount of activity in the deeper, oldest and most primitive part of the brain (the limbic system) increases. Thus we stop thinking and we start feeling that primordial dimension of ourselves. The limbic system is partly subconscious and this explains the involuntary contractions, vocalizations and laughter that often happen at, and just after, climax.

Dopamine is released from the brain when you eat a delicious piece of chocolate, puff on a cigarette (if you are addicted to nicotine) or when you drink alcohol, but the highs produced from these triggers of dopamine release, do not compare to the intensity of that produced during an orgasm. No wonder that people who cannot have a fulfilling sexual relationship are more likely to become addicted to unhealthy triggers of dopamine release. It's not surprising that an exciting sexual relationship can help people to lose weight or overcome unhealthy addictions. We have all seen people lose a lot of weight when they fall in love!

You may think that this sounds good enough, but wait it gets even better, because for most people the joy of sex does not end abruptly after an orgasm. The afterglow of sex produces a relaxed, romantic, affectionate and trusting feeling. Many people find themselves laughing and cuddling and free of fear and inhibition after an orgasm. These warm loving feelings towards your partner are produced by the release of the hormone oxytocin from your brain. The more you cuddle, touch, caress and kiss your partner the more oxytocin is released into your body. In particular, the stimulation of your erogenous zones in the nipples and genital organs causes more oxytocin to be released. No wonder we love songs that say "Do it to me one more time, I can never get enough of a man like you oh oh."

When we are at the pinnacle of an orgasm (the climax) our body is flooded with high levels of oxytocin and this leads to involuntary muscular contractions of the uterus, vagina and pelvic floor. Multiple orgasms release even more dopamine and oxytocin and the pleasure intensifies.

The afterglow of sexual orgasm is really produced by oxytocin and it is very powerful as a bonding hormone, helping you to make a deep emotional attachment to your lover. You become more trusting, less fearful and feel secure and content. For these reasons oxytocin has been dubbed *the snuggle hormone*. The effects of oxytocin are not short lived and, not only does it help you to fall in love, it helps you to stay in love. We all crave security and love and, for most women, that desire is greater than the desire for the short lived climax. If you have regular sex with your partner the recurrent release of oxytocin keeps you bonded and attached to your partner. Oxytocin helps couples stay together physically and emotionally.

Help for orgasms

No matter where you fall in the *normal spectrum* of sexual response, you can improve your orgasms. Indeed with the right technique from your partner or from yourself via masturbation, you may be able to achieve some multiple orgasms.

The vast majority of women masturbate; they will use either their fingers or a vibrator. This is quite healthy and normal and is not a sign of any character weakness or sexual depravity. Masturbation will not lead to any increase in diseases of the vulva and pelvic organs.

Regular orgasms achieved through masturbation may be healthy and promote a better circulation of blood to the pelvic organs and strengthen the pelvic floor muscles.

Many normal women begin to masturbate during their teen years and this way they get to know themselves and can avoid having sexual intercourse before they are ready and before they have adequate contraception. Some women do not begin to explore the feeling of masturbation and clitoral stimulation until much later in life, say in their late 20s or 30s. In these women it is often an incompetent or selfish lover that leaves them frustrated and wondering "Is this all there is?" - that prompts them to masturbate. The orgasm they give themselves will relieve their sexual frustration.

Many women will need help to orgasm, especially as they get older, if they have hormonal imbalances or if they have health problems. The sex hormones estrogen, progesterone and testosterone prepare and prime your genital organs for sex. They make you interested and ready to receive. Low levels of estrogen cause the vulva and vagina to thin and shrink (atrophy) and their membranes dry out. This makes you too fragile for sex.

Adequate levels of all three sex hormones keep your vagina and vulva robust, plumper, supple and moist – they make you responsive and inviting. They also increase blood flow to the vulva and increase sensitivity. Testosterone makes you the warrior woman and gives you the confidence and desire to conquer the man in your life – at least in bed that is, but it can also promote emotional strength as well.

Hormonal creams and oxytocin can make a huge difference and can turn the vast majority of women of all ages into orgasmic creatures. At the very least, we can bring back your sex drive and promote great enjoyment of sex. See our treatment section which explains how to use these things.

You need to be a good communicator with your sex partner and, if you feel frustrated, tell your partner the exact technique you need them to use for you to achieve satisfaction. If poor communication is a persistent problem, consult a professional sex therapist together.

Sexual desire

The desire for sex is often called *libido* and this varies tremendously between women. Some women have a continual interest in sex and are always ready for their partner. Other women do not think about sex very much and are more focused on their career, children or family.

Sexual desire generally reduces with age although older women often find that hormone replacement therapy can rekindle their interest. It is quite normal for libido to be higher at the beginning of a new relationship. Once you get to know each other, and have conquered your mate so to speak, the intensity of sexual desire may gradually wane.

Your environment has a big effect upon your libido and women often find that their libido resurfaces like the Phoenix when they go away with their partner on a holiday away from family and work. Yes, you need more holidays together!

Some women have a naturally low libido and this does not worry them; in other words low libido is not an issue or a medical problem, unless it worries you.

Sexual desire in women is often affected by the physical and mental status of their partner. If your partner smells like a brewery, or an ashtray, is drug affected, has body odor, or is grumpy, well, then reading a magazine or eating an apple pie with ice cream has got to be sexier than sex!

Let's face it — we want to feel special if our partner wants to have sex with us — we are worth their effort!

3. What are the causes of poor libido in women?

Declining levels of sex hormone production with age

One day, a patient came to see me all the way from a small country town called Lightening Ridge in North Western New South Wales. She had travelled over 300 miles on a bus to get to my medical office in Sydney. She was of peri-menopausal age and had recently married a man several years younger; this was likely to present challenges for her, as her hormones were waning at this age. I asked her "How can I help you?" She made me chuckle when she replied "Oh Doctor Cabot you are my last resort, as my doctor does not have a clue how to help me!"

I replied "Well, what did you tell your doctor?" She exclaimed "I told him that I have lost all my lib-ee-dooo and I want it back!" I thought to myself - "No wonder her local country doctor could not help her, as he had probably never heard of the disease 'lost lib-ee-dooo.' "What she meant to express to her doctor is that she had lost her libido or desire for sex! Of course quite a few country doctors think that when women reach a certain age (maybe over 45) that they do not need a libido or a healthy sex life. Young doctors may be guilty of this as-sumption too, as they may view all women over 40 as *old*.

This patient was very relieved when I told her that I could restore her sexual desire and ability to have orgasms by giving her a cream containing bio-identical hormones. This cream is made up by a com-pounding chemist to the exact recipe in the prescription which is de-signed by the prescribing doctor to match the patient's blood tests and symptoms.

I designed a cream containing bio-identical estrogen and proges-terone and another cream containing testosterone for this lady. She went back on the bus to Lightening Ridge full of expectation that she would rediscover her lost lib-ee-dooo!

A compounding pharmacy in Sydney would make up her prescription and mail the hormone creams to her Post Office Box in Lightening Ridge. I have a little saying "You know when you have reached a certain age when your sex hormones arrive via parcel in the mail". This prescription really worked, as when the patient returned for her follow up consult 6 months later, she said "Oh Dr Cabot I have had the strongest and best orgasm I have had in 20 years!"

At one of the medical centers where I consult, I share a little joke with the secretaries who are all females of a certain age. We all came up with the unsexiest thing you can think of – and we decided it was a turnip. If you feel like a turnip when it comes to sex, then you probably have the sex hormone levels of a turnip – in other words very very low. We then coined the term *turnip's disease* to describe how one feels when all their sex hormones disappear.

When patients would phone up for their hormone level test results, if they were all very low, we would say to the patient, "You have turnip's disease." The patient would respond, "Oh, that sounds very serious!" Once we explained what it meant, they would burst into peals of laughter and say "Yes, that's how I feel, about as sexy as a dried up turnip!" Two of the secretaries had T-shirts made up with a printed logo of *Turnips*. It sounds a little crazy but it gave us plenty of giggles.

After menopause, most women lose adequate production of estrogen and progesterone and this may reduce sexual desire and the ability to enjoy sex. The loss of estrogen causes the tissues of the vagina and vulva to shrink and dry out and the clitoris becomes smaller and less sensitive. Indeed, the clitoris may become tender to touch so that foreplay becomes uncomfortable. The loss of estrogen causes a loss of vaginal secretions. The loss of progesterone causes a reduced sexual desire and may also cause mood changes.

After menopause, the amount of testosterone produced by the ovaries and fat tissues varies a lot and this is why blood tests to measure the level of testosterone are so important to choose the types and amounts of hormones required in the cream. Some women produce plenty of testosterone after menopause and thus do not need any testosterone in their prescription. Other women may need testosterone in their prescription if their blood tests show low levels.

Testosterone is a very important hormone for libido and sexual response and, in women with low levels, it is essential to prescribe some natural testosterone, either in the form of a cream or lozenge. Testosterone can make women more sexually assertive and sexually confident and indeed too much testosterone can result in excessive sexual drive in some women.

Menopause

The human female is the only creature known to live much longer than her sex glands and reproductive capacity; in this context we are very different to men so no wonder us older girls need a little help to keep up in the bedroom.

When our ovaries run out of eggs, (follicles) our production of progesterone ceases completely and our estrogen levels become very low. The average age of menopause is 50 years but a significant percentage of women go through an early menopause and their eggs are totally gone before they get to 40 – this is called a premature menopause. I have had patients who go through menopause in their 20s and these women need a lot more help with hormone replacement.

Before the menopause, the majority of our estrogen is produced by our ovaries. After the menopause, when the ovaries are devoid of useful eggs, the vast majority of our estrogen is produced away from our ovaries in our fat tissue. I have found that thinner women often have more pronounced estrogen deficiency symptoms.

The blood test for menopause is a measurement of the Follicle Stimulating Hormone (FSH) and if this is elevated you are menopausal and you have no fertile eggs. If your FSH levels are over 30 IU/L on two separate blood tests, you are deemed menopausal and the higher your FSH levels, the lower your estrogen and progesterone levels will be. The FSH is produced by the pituitary gland and acts to stimulate the ovaries back into production of the sex hormones estrogen and progesterone. In post menopausal women it is not uncommon to see very high levels of FSH around 100 to 200 IU/L, which are coming from the pituitary gland and this means your estrogen levels will be very low. These high levels of FSH will not be successful in stimulating your ovaries back to work because they no longer have any eggs left in them to respond to the FSH. Your ovaries have *closed shop* or *gone on strike* forever and thus these high levels of FSH achieve nothing but do serve as an accurate blood test for menopause.

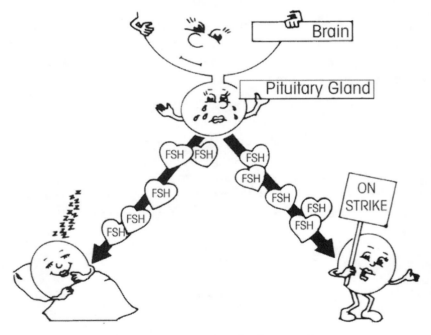

Menopausal Ovaries

All women want to know if they are truly menopausal and need to know their FSH level to determine this. If your FSH level is very high, you have no fertile eggs and will no longer have to worry about contraception – this may improve your libido! If you are taking the oral contraceptive pill, you will need to stop taking it for several months before having a blood test for menopause; otherwise the test will be inaccurate. So don't waste your money having blood tests for your hormone levels while you are still taking the oral contraceptive pill. Many doctors do not realize this so it's wise to inform yourself.

Progesterone deficiency

Progesterone is a sex hormone that is made by the female ovaries during the latter half of the menstrual cycle and in vast amounts by the placenta during pregnancy. Many women start to become progesterone deficient in their late 30s and 40s, way before they get to menopause. By the time these women get to menopause their levels may only be 20% of their youthful progesterone levels.

Progesterone has anti-ageing properties and is important for sex drive. Progesterone exerts a calming effect and can promote emotional contentment and stability. The brain has receptors for progesterone and this is why natural hormones can be so beneficial for emotional disorders.

If you find that your mood and sex drive lowers during the one to two weeks before your menstrual bleeding commences, then you will probably benefit from natural progesterone.

Progesterone deficiency is very common in women today because they often delay pregnancy to later in life and have fewer pregnancies. Progesterone deficiency can cause unpleasant moods such as anxiety, irritability, irrational thinking, poor libido and depression. Progesterone deficiency can also cause physical health problems such as heavy and/or painful menstrual bleeding, endometriosis, fibroids, increased risk of cancer, premenstrual headaches, polycystic ovarian syndrome and unexplained infertility.

The use of natural progesterone was first advocated back in the 1960s by Dr. Katharina Dalton, an English physician who was somewhat of a 'PMS Guru'.

Natural progesterone can be very useful in reducing the following problems-

- Depression, anxiety, and mood changes
- Iron deficiency and fatigue
- Heavy menstrual bleeding
- Menstrual pain
- Pelvic congestion, pain and bloating
- Breast pain
- Poor libido
- Insomnia

It is important to realize that Dr. Dalton recommended the use of *natural* progesterone, which has a chemical structure identical to the progesterone produced by the ovaries. Natural progesterone is made in the laboratory from the plant hormone called diosgenin found in soybeans and sweet potatoes (yams). Because natural progesterone is identical to the progesterone produced by the ovaries it is called a *bio-identical hormone.*

Unfortunately, doctors often prescribe strong synthetic brands of progesterone called 'progestogens', mistakenly believing that they will have the same effect as natural progesterone. This is not true and synthetic progesterone will usually make most of the symptoms of PMS much worse.

Many of these synthetic progestogens are derived from male (testosterone-like) synthetic hormones and so may cause side effects such as increased appetite, depression, irritability, weight gain, fluid retention, acne, greasy skin and increased cholesterol. These synthetic progestogen hormones attach onto the natural progesterone receptors found throughout the body and brain, but they cannot switch on all these receptors.

Only natural progesterone can turn on ALL the progesterone receptors just as a key turns and releases a lock. So you can understand that synthetic progestogens will not have the same beneficial effect as natural progesterone and indeed many women feel more depressed and tired when they take them. However, synthetic progestogens are effective at reducing heavy menstrual bleeding and some types of gynecological problems such as endometriosis.

Progesterone deficiency is common in:

• Young women with menstrual problems
• Women after childbirth where it is associated with postnatal depression
• Women with cyclical mood disorders and bipolar illness
• Women with thyroid problems such as Hashimoto's thyroiditis or Grave's disease
• Women after miscarriage
• Peri-menopausal women

How do I know if I am progesterone deficient?

It is not generally necessary or useful to do blood or salivary tests to prove that a deficiency of progesterone exists. This is because a doctor who understands progesterone can tell from the history of the patient if they are deficient. Keeping a menstrual calendar of symptoms to show your doctor can help to pinpoint the premenstrual exacerbation.

Symptoms of progesterone deficiency include:

• Heavy and/or painful periods
• Poor libido
• Insomnia
• Premenstrual headaches
• Fibroids, endometriosis or adenomyosis of the uterus
• Unexplained infertility
• Polycystic ovarian syndrome
• Premenstrual syndrome/moodiness and postnatal depression
• Iron deficiency

- Infrequent or irregular periods
- Hair loss
- Breast pain and/or lumpiness

The good news is that natural progesterone therapy can often alleviate these symptoms in women of all ages. Thus one would think that natural progesterone is commonly prescribed for these diverse and common problems.

In reality however, few doctors prescribe natural progesterone because it cannot be patented by drug companies. Thus drug companies do not promote it or educate doctors about its use or benefits. This is a pity and results in much unneeded suffering for women.

In my opinion, the best way to administer natural progesterone is in the form of a cream which is rubbed into the skin. See Treatment Section page 50.

Polycystic ovarian syndrome

Georgina came to my medical practice one day as a new patient and her story has really stuck in my mind. She plonked herself in the chair on the other side of my desk and looked tired and distraught. I asked her "Why have you come to see me today? She replied "I am sick of lying in bed at night and thinking of 27 ways to kill my husband". Unfortunately, she was not joking and had really come to the end of the road, so to speak. I think she saw me as the last resort and thankfully I was able to relieve her suffering.

Georgina had all the classic symptoms of polycystic ovarian syndrome (PCOS) – she was overweight, apple shaped (android body type), hated sex and had not had a menstrual period for 2 years. She was aged 39 so her lack of regular menstrual bleeding was abnormal, considering she was not menopausal.

Blood tests on Georgina revealed that her levels of male hormones (androgens) were very high and her progesterone levels were very low. She also had high blood levels of insulin and was pre-diabetic.

Georgina had been on anti-depressant drugs for 2 years and they were no longer controlling her depression and aggressive moods. This poor lady had hormones more like that of a man than a woman and really needed progesterone.

I prescribed natural progesterone cream 100mg daily and 2 weeks later Georgina had a menstrual bleed – for the first time in 2 years!

With the onset of the bleeding came an emotional release and a feeling of calm relaxation. I also prescribed a low carbohydrate diet free of grains and sugar and told her to follow the eating plan in my book *Fatty Liver – You Can Reverse It*. Georgina had a fatty liver caused from the high insulin levels due to her previously high carbohydrate diet. Her poor liver function had contributed to her hormonal imbalance, so I also prescribed a supplement of Livatone Plus and selenium to support her liver function.

Over the next 6 months, Georgina continued to have a regular monthly menstrual cycle and lost her feelings of aggression and irritability. She felt calm and content and lost a considerable amount of weight. Her facial hair and acne also improved greatly and her sex drive returned. Luckily for her poor unsuspecting husband she no longer fantasized about ways to kill him!

Hormonal imbalances can drive women to do all sorts of extreme things, especially premenstrually and during the postnatal period, and these things can be most out of character.

Dr Katharina Dalton dedicated her life to helping women with PMS and postnatal depression and she was really the pioneer of natural progesterone therapy and wrote several books on the subject. Dr Dalton acted as an expert witness in criminal court cases trying to have the charges against women mitigated because of their hormonal problems. She managed to prove that in many cases natural progesterone therapy could have prevented aggressive behavior.

Fatigue

Lack of energy is a common cause of disinterest in sex because having sex takes time and effort, especially if you are to do it well and enjoy it. If you are too tired it is easy to understand that you would rather use the precious time to rest or sleep.

Common causes of fatigue in women are iron deficiency, depression, lack of sleep and the excessive busyness of being a mother, domestic goddess and bread winner. Poor diet, lack of exercise and general poor health produce fatigue, which can drain away our sexual energy.

Many women tell me that if they go away on a holiday just with their husband their libido returns and they enjoy fulfilling sex. Life is just too busy and complicated these days for many women to have the luxury of time and peace to be conscious of their sexuality.

Stress

I see many women who have to spend most of their life caring for others. They may have elderly or sick parents, children with disabilities or behavioral problems, or a husband with his own mental and emotional issues. Women tend to be the problem solvers and rescuers and, in doing this, they often lose themselves. These angels often deserve a medal of honor and I take my hat off to them every day. Hopefully we can all be more aware of the sacrifices they make and enable them to have more respite.

Depression

The symptoms of depression often manifest as fatigue, loss of enjoyment and loss of interest in life and may insidiously develop over several years. Obviously this can impair your emotional relationship with your partner.

Depression is more common during the first 12 months after childbirth, when it is called postnatal depression, and around the time of menopause. Depression is often associated with feelings of low self esteem and poor self image and loss of interest in the opposite sex. Depression is the result of a chemical imbalance in the brain with reduced levels of the brain's neurotransmitters – namely dopamine, serotonin and adrenalin.

Modern day anti-depressants are effective at restoring the brain's levels of these neurotransmitters and, once they are back to normal, the symptoms of depression disappear. Anti-depressants may improve your emotional relationship with your partner, which may help your low libido, however some anti-depressant medications make it impossible to achieve an orgasm. In this case oxytocin nasal spray and natural hormone creams may help a lot.

The oral contraceptive pill

The oral contraceptive pill (OCP) comes in two forms. The most common form is called the combined oral contraceptive pill and contains estrogen combined with progesterone. The other form is known as the progesterone only pill because it does not contain any estrogen. The combined oral contraceptive pill prevents over 99% of pregnancies and the progesterone only pill is less effective as a contraceptive preventing around 95% of pregnancies. Both types of oral contraceptive pills contain synthetic hormones, as natural hormones are not strong enough to prevent pregnancy.

The synthetic hormones in the contraceptive pill must be broken down (metabolized) by the liver and this process stimulates the liver to make greater amounts of a protein called Sex Hormone Binding Globulin (SHBG). SHBG acts to bind the naturally produced sex hormones in the body especially testosterone. Once a hormone is bound or attached to SHBG it is not free to act in the body and is thus inactivated. This reduction in the amounts of free testosterone available to the body often reduces the sex drive because testosterone exerts a stimulating effect on the sex drive.

It is not uncommon for women to complain of loss of sex drive after they have been on the contraceptive pill for several months and this lowering of free testosterone is the main reason. The SHBG also binds the circulating levels of estrogen and this can result in vaginal dryness.

The progesterone only mini pill is less likely to reduce the sex drive than the combined oral contraceptive pill. If you are on the contraceptive pill and find that it has reduced your sex drive or caused vaginal dryness, this can be helped by applying to the vulva a cream combining natural estrogen and natural testosterone. This cream needs to be used on a regular basis.

Possible side effects of the OCP include-

- Migraine headaches, which can be severe
- Nausea and gallstones
- Fluid retention
- Weight gain and bloating
- Reduced or total loss of sex drive
- Breast pain and lumpiness
- Blood clots and aggravation of varicose veins
- Elevation of blood pressure
- Moodiness and depression in susceptible women

If the OCP gives you side effects, you will need to experiment with your doctor to try different brands of the OCP, as they contain different types of hormones. All the hormones used in the OCP are synthetic and some women will be unable to tolerate the side effects.

In women with heavy menstrual bleeding, a contraceptive intra-uterine device called the Mirena can work effectively to reduce the menstrual bleeding to very light amounts. The Mirena does not usually help to overcome PMS symptoms such as mood disorders and low libido and, in such cases, the natural progesterone cream can be used with the Mirena. This is quite safe and does not interfere with the contraceptive efficiency of the Mirena.

Note*: It is imperative that women who wish to avoid pregnancy and are taking drugs or hormones to treat low libido, sexual problems or PMS have adequate means of contraception.*

When a woman is taking the oral contraceptive pill, blood tests to measure the natural levels of sex hormones are not useful or meaningful, as all they will show is that you are on the pill and that you have high levels of SHBG and low levels of estrogen and testosterone.

If the OCP is destroying your libido, try an alternative method of contraception that will not reduce your sex hormones as much — for example the progestogen implant known as Implanon or the Depot Provera injection. Some women find that a MIRENA intrauterine contraceptive device suits them well, as it lightens the amount of menstrual bleeding and does not reduce their own natural hormone levels.

Medications that reduce sexual desire

Many medications can interfere with sex drive and sexual function but are unlikely to be the sole cause of these problems. The disease for which you are taking the medication may also be reducing your sexual function and it can be difficult to know what percentage of the problem is caused by the medications compared to the disease. If you suspect a medication has reduced your sex drive, talk to your doctor as there are alternative medications that you can take for your disease that will not affect your sex life.

The following medications can reduce sex drive:

• Drugs that affect the brain's levels of serotonin and/or dopamine
• Drugs that increase Sex Hormone Binding Globulin (such as oral estrogens and the oral contraceptive pill)
• Drugs that reduce the action of testosterone such as cyproterone acetate
• Some commonly prescribed antacids

The most common drugs known to reduce sex drive and orgasmic ability are anti-depressant medications. Antipsychotic medications used for the treatment of schizophrenia or bipolar illness can reduce sex drive. Blood pressure medications (anti-hypertensives) can also reduce sexual function.

I should mention here that the mineral magnesium in a dose of 400mg daily can lower blood pressure and improve sexual function in both sexes. For information on natural therapies for depression see my book *Help for Depression and Anxiety.*

It is interesting to note that cholesterol lowering drugs, especially if taken in high doses, can reduce sex drive and function in both sexes. This may not only be due to the direct effects of these drugs on the tissues and nerves, but also because the body makes all its natural sex hormones from cholesterol. Very low cholesterol levels often mean very low sex hormone levels. I am not a fan of very low cholesterol levels – see my book *Cholesterol the Real Truth – are the drugs you take making you sick?*

Do not stop any medications that you are taking without talking to your doctor first. But do talk to your doctor, as you may be much better on a lower dose or a different brand of drug.

Vaginal odor and infection

Vaginal odor can be a turn off for both partners of a sexual relationship just as much as bad breath can be; interestingly, by improving your gut health you can improve both problems. Vaginal odor is most often caused by unfriendly bacteria such as streptococci or Ecoli growing in the vagina and these can originate on the skin around the anus and from the bowel. This condition is called Bacterial Vaginosis (BV).

By strengthening your immune system using the strategies on page 75 you will reduce these unfriendly vaginal bacteria.

Infection with the yeast organism called candida does not usually produce an odor but often causes an excess vaginal discharge that is thick and white and may cause itchiness around the vulva.

All these infections can be controlled by improving your immune system and your diet. Try to eat more raw vegetable salads and avoid all sugar. Sugar feeds bacterial and yeast infections and you should eliminate processed foods as well as foods high in sugar. Use natural low carbohydrate sweeteners instead of sugar, such as stevia, erythritol, xylitol or chicory root.

Avoid antibiotic drugs and antibiotic creams if you can, as these will only produce a temporary fix and lead to an overgrowth of candida. Many doctors prescribe strong antibiotic creams such as Dalacin V or strong antifungal drugs such as Diflucan, which I am not in favour of, as they can be toxic to the liver especially if used repetitively.

One harmless treatment for candida is the use of vaginal pessaries containing boric acid in a dose of 600mg per pessary which is used for 14 days. Another very useful and harmless treatment is to douche the vagina with a weak solution of tea tree oil.

The company called Thursday Plantation makes a feminine hygiene gel which is mixed with warm sterile water (boil the water first to sterilize it). Mix the gel with the appropriate amount of water as per the label instructions and fill the douche balloon with this. Lie in an empty bath and place the douche nozzle in the vagina and flush the solution into the vaginal cavity. This will flush out the excess mucus within the vagina in which the bacteria and candida live.

Tea tree oil is effective against bacteria, candida and other yeasts and will prevent them from growing and thus causing the odor. The tea tree oil has a cleansing fresh fragrance and if the gel solution is mixed with the correct amount of water, as per the label instructions, it will not be irritating.

Some doctors are against douching as they believe it is not natural or physiological to use this practice. I think it is much safer than using strong antibiotics and antifungal drugs.

Another useful technique is to insert a tablespoon of plain unflavored Greek Style yogurt into the vagina every day as this will populate the vagina with friendly bacteria which will compete with the unfriendly smelly bacteria. Yogurt keeps the vagina more acidic which reduces infections.

A pro biotic formula can also be swallowed daily to improve the gut flora.

Herpes

Genital herpes is caused by infection with the herpes simplex virus (HSV) and is a very common problem which can really put a dampener on your sex life.

The initial infection of HSV is often very dramatic with widespread blisters on the vulva. These are painful and often associated with fever and aches and pains. Some women suffer with further recurrent attacks of genital herpes and this varies from once a month to once in every blue moon.

The antiviral drug called Acyclovir works very well and reduces symptoms and shortens the time the blisters are present. Other effective antiviral drugs are available such as Valacyclovir and Famciclovir and the earlier you take these drugs the better they work.

If you have recurrent herpes keep a supply of these antiviral drugs at home. If you are experiencing very frequent recurrent attacks of herpes, you can take Acyclovir everyday to suppress the virus so you do not get any blisters or other symptoms; this also reduces viral shedding from infected areas, thus reducing transmission to your partner. Condoms prevent transmission to your partner.

It is vital to avoid excessive stress, as this will weaken your immune system leading to more frequent attacks, although long term Acyclovir can prevent this. I have found that patients with recurrent herpes benefit greatly by taking a selenium and zinc supplement, such as Selenomune powder. Selenium and zinc are minerals which help your cellular immune system to fight viruses. I call selenium the *viral birth control pill* because it reduces the ability of viruses to replicate and thus keeps them in a low inactive state. If you keep getting frequent attacks of herpes it is vital to follow a plan to strengthen your entire immune system and this will gradually reduce the frequency and severity of herpes attacks. Follow the plan on page 75.

Vaginismus

The term vaginismus describes the involuntary spasm of the muscles in and around the vagina when entry of the vagina is attempted during sexual activity or a pelvic examination. The strength of the muscular contractions can be very high so that entry of the vagina is impossible and this can cause extreme discomfort for the man and the woman. The most common cause of vaginismus is anxiety and fear, perhaps of the unknown, or perhaps stimulated by the memory of rape or sexual abuse.

Another possible cause of vaginismus is a physical abnormality in the pelvic cavity and vagina such as pelvic infection, bladder infection or endometriosis. These problems may cause pain on attempted entry of the vagina and this may lead to protective muscle spasm. It is vital to see a specialist gynecologist for a pelvic exam (if possible) or a pelvic ultrasound scan at the very least; these tests will exclude physical causes of vaginal spasm and pain.

Once diagnosed, vaginismus is best treated by a professional sex therapist, who may be a doctor or psychologist; they will use counselling, relaxation exercises and perhaps even some hypnosis. Hypnotherapy can be very effective. It is vital to work on improving self confidence and self esteem. The sex therapist will often need to teach you how to use vaginal dilators to relax and desensitize your vaginal tissues; these work very well although a total cure may take several years. This is something that cannot be rushed and must be done at your own pace.

Regular exercises, yoga and Pilates may also help a lot. A magnesium supplement will help to relax your nervous system and your muscles.

Pain in the area of the vulva

Some women suffer with a chronic or recurrent discomfort in the lips and/or vestibule of the vulva – this problem is called vulvodynia. It is very uncomfortable and may feel like a dull ache, a burning stinging feeling, a pressure, rawness and an itch or a combination of all these sensations. It is usually associated with painful sexual intercourse.

The cause is somewhat mysterious and variable and has been put down to dysfunctional nerve endings in the vulva or nerve injury. The vulva, and especially the part known as the vestibule, contains a huge amount of dense nerve fibers and, if these are dysfunctional, then it's no wonder that severe chronic pain can persist. If the vestibule is touched by a doctor or a sexual partner, even very lightly, it feels painful. Many sufferers find it is impossible to use tampons, and sexual intercourse may be painful or impossible. Often women with vulvodynia have never enjoyed sex because of this pain and they seek to avoid it.

So what causes the nerve pain? There have been many theories put forward and the most logical is chronic inflammation in the nerve endings and/or in the skin of the vulva; in most cases one cannot see this inflammation on a physical examination of the vulva; thus it is microscopic. Women with vulvodynia are more likely to have chronic inflammation in the bladder wall and this is called interstitial cystitis which causes painful and frequent urination.

If you have vulvodynia it is important to see a gynecologist who specializes in this area – for more information see resources section at the end of this book.

The specialist doctor will rule out diseases, which could masquerade as vulvodynia but need a different treatment. These diseases include skin diseases such as eczema, lichen planus, lichen sclerosis, contact dermatitis, autoimmune diseases and infections. A general practitioner may miss or misdiagnose these disorders.

The treatment of vulvodynia will take time and can be very successful if you are persistent and patient. The most important thing is to reduce the inflammation that is causing the pain in the nerves and the skin and this is best achieved by following my immune strategies on page 75. These strategies work because they are treating the cause, although it may take 6 to 12 months to get this inflammation completely under control.

Other treatments can be tried such as a topical anesthetic gel (such as Xylocaine) applied to the painful areas, especially if you want to attempt sexual intercourse. Cortisone creams reduce inflammation by suppressing it and can be used for flare ups; however, try to avoid daily long term use. Castor oil and zinc cream (used for diaper rash) can be very soothing and protective of the thin skin of the vestibule.

If you have a lot of stress and anxiety, try a strong magnesium supplement such as Magnesium Ultrapotent powder to calm the central nervous system and the nerves in the vulva.

In highly stressed women who cannot sleep, the use of a low dose of a tricyclic anti-depressant can greatly dull the pain and at least you will get a proper deep sleep. I emphasize the use of a *tiny* dose of a tricyclic anti-depressant to be used initially; then you will not get any side effects such as sedation and constipation. These small doses can be made up by a compounding pharmacist.

Urinary tract infections

In some women sexual activity aggravates a tendency to urinary tract infections. The urethra is very close to the opening of the vagina so it is easy to understand how thrusting of the penis could push bacteria up into the urethra or for the urethra to become traumatized and irritated.

You may have heard of *honeymoon cystitis* which is an acute bladder infection following a night of passionate love making. It's a sure way to ruin your honeymoon!

If you are prone to recurrent urinary tract infections or interstitial cystitis, follow the strategies on page 75 to strengthen your immune system. This will prevent most urinary tract infections, as well as gradually overcome interstitial cystitis. Take extra vitamin C every day in a dose of 1000 to 3000mg.

Prolapse of the pelvic floor and/or vagina

Some women feel that their vagina is too large and they cannot control the muscles around their vagina. This is common after multiple childbirths and it produces an inability to contract the vaginal muscles around the penis and often reduces sensitivity.

In such cases, ask your doctor to refer you to a physiotherapist who can teach you pelvic floor exercises. This often works extremely well and you can practise these exercises whilst driving, washing the dishes or watching TV. It will give you much better control of your bladder as well and often overcomes urinary incontinence. Such physiotherapists have machines that electrically stimulate the vaginal and pelvic floor muscles which teach you which muscles you need to strengthen. It is always worth going to a physiotherapist who specializes in this area.

In some women the walls of the vagina start to descend outside the vaginal opening and you can feel these bulges at the front or back of your vagina. This is called a prolapse and if it becomes worse it may drag down the lower part of your bladder and rectum. You may feel embarrassed about this and it can interfere with bladder and bowel control. A good gynecologist can easily repair these prolapses via vaginal surgery and tighten the vagina at the same time by removing the excess and floppy tissues. You will be brand new again with a smaller vagina and no prolapse.

Constipation

If you are constipated, feces can accumulate in the rectum and you may feel this when the penis pushes backwards in your vagina and this may make it hard for you to relax.

To overcome constipation, pelvic floor exercises can help and so can yoga and Pilates. Drink more water and increase the amount of raw vegetables and fruits in the diet. Use a gluten free fiber such as Fibertone Powder and take 2 tablespoons of ground flaxseeds daily.

Poor circulation of blood to the vulva

The sexual response and orgasm requires a large amount of blood to flow into the vulva and vaginal blood vessels and if this does not occur it will be much harder to become lubricated and to orgasm. There are factors that can reduce this circulation of blood, such as diabetes, smoking and high blood pressure.

To improve the circulation of blood we can take various nutritional supplements and we need to take them regularly. The most important one to take is magnesium, and the powder called Magnesium Ultrapotent provides 400mg of highly absorbed magnesium in one teaspoon. It has a pleasant flavor, being sweetened with stevia, and works quickly, usually within 20 minutes.

Vitamin C helps to improve the health of the arteries and I recommend you take 1000mg daily. Liquid fish oil is of great benefit to improve the circulation of blood and I recommend you purchase a good brand and keep it refrigerated. Take the recommended dose on the label, although if your circulation is very poor you may need a higher dose, which is quite safe to take.

4. The Search for Love

Love is the most wonderful feeling you can experience and I have observed that we seek that feeling in our lives at many levels, both conscious and subconscious.

When we are young we usually seek love from our parents and then once our hormones kick in, we seek it from our lovers. As we age, most of us come to realize that the feeling of love exists within us and we try to connect with that inner buzz that makes us feel satisfied and peaceful.

To feel love is a craving that never leaves us and, even though it is so close and exists within us, for many people it seems so far away. Sometimes we just don't know how to tap into it, however there are simple meditation techniques we can learn to achieve this. It is very practical and effective and I was fortunate to learn how to do this when I was only 21 years of age. Let me tell you they did not teach these techniques at medical school!

Let me tell you of a few case histories, which to me illustrate the eternal quest for love.

One of my long term patients is a delightful lady who, by conventional standards, is very eccentric. She is physically attractive and suffers with bipolar illness, which has made her life a series of highs and lows. Her bipolar illness was not diagnosed or treated effectively until she was in her forties. After commencing an anti-depressant medication she discovered a normal and happy emotional state, which had unfortunately eluded her for most of her difficult life.

She had been sexually abused as a very young child and possibly as an infant by her alcoholic father. This had totally screwed up her sexuality and femininity so much so that she had never had normal sexual relations with a man. This did not worry her on a conscious level, as all she craved was to feel normal and not to be plagued by the crazy thoughts in her head.

She had etched out a living as a psychic and in this she was gifted, having helped many people. When she was on an emotional high she worked hard as a psychic and received reasonable money from her grateful clients; but she still never managed to settle down. When she became depressed she withdrew from others and lived on the road in her car. It was an awful and hard existence and she came to accept that this series of highs and lows was normal for her.

She presented to the outside world as an attractive and happy person, able to inspire and help other people, but deep down inside she was frightened and sad.

She was fortunate to meet a caring and clever psychiatrist who diagnosed her with bipolar illness and treated her with the correct medications. These medications enabled her to see what a terrible and miserable state she had been trapped in for most of her life. She told me that it was such a huge relief to discover that she could feel calm and stable and in control of her life and that she did not know how she had managed to survive all these years living like a frightened animal in her car.

Such is the miracle of modern day psychiatric drugs that can free a human being from the misery of mental and emotional illness.

This woman had never had children, as she had never been able to have normal sexual relations with men after her terrible sexual abuse. She had also suffered with severe endometriosis and bladder problems, which had necessitated a hysterectomy. In spite of her surgery she continued to have major problems with control of her bladder possibly as a result of physical trauma caused by sexual abuse.

During her last visit to me she told me that for the first time in her life she was interested in meeting a nice man and becoming intimate with him. It was obvious to me that she was ready to seek love and affection. It had taken this woman more than forty years to feel comfortable and confident enough to seek a deep relationship with a man.

I am really looking forward to seeing her again and hope that she can meet a caring man worthy of her physical and spiritual beauty. In the past, her self esteem had been rock bottom and she told me that she felt dirty and damaged because her body had been used and debased just like that of an animal by her father. This story is a testimony to the ability of the human spirit to be healed by the help of good medicine and compassion.

The need to be loved is such a strong subconscious desire and, if not fulfilled, many physical and emotional symptoms can manifest in our lives.

This was illustrated by a woman who came to see me with an array of physical problems that had been put down to adrenal gland exhaustion. She was very fatigued and had aches and pains typical of fibromyalgia where one feels tender and stiff in the muscles.

She spent a full hour telling me about her symptoms and during this time she kept referring to her mother with whom she had a difficult relationship. Her mother was closer to her two sisters and tended to be critical of her, so much so, that her mother would often exclude her from family gatherings. This woman really craved for time and attention from her mother and yet she felt unaccepted by her mother.

She sought her mother's love and approval but she felt continually unable to get this. I found it fascinating that, in between her detailed discussion of her physical symptoms, she kept referring back to her mother, as I had never asked her about her mother and I was focused on diagnosing the cause of her fibromyalgia.

At the end of the consultation this patient started crying, although at no stage had I asked her any emotional questions. This led me to say to her "By the way, do you realize how beautiful you are?" She replied "What?" This may sound rather incongruous for a medical consultation, but it just came out of me spontaneously because I could see the beauty and purity in the pathos of this woman, seeking approval and love from her obviously screwed up mother.

This woman felt unwell because she was unloved – it was not adrenal exhaustion, it was love exhaustion. I reaffirmed that she was a beautiful and expressive lady and that she would respond to counselling to improve her self esteem. I also encouraged her to learn to meditate to get to know herself so she could really learn to love and approve of herself. Instead of seeking her mother's approval she would be better served by seeking her own approval.

We ended the consult with a hug and I referred her to a good psychologist. I also treated her fibromyalgia with magnesium and omega 3 fatty acids – after all I am a holistic doctor, although in her case, I suspected that my caring remark would have a more therapeutic effect.

5. Lubricants

Vaginal lubricants are often needed in the following cases –

- Low estrogen levels
- Women on the oral contraceptive pill
- Women with skin problems of the vulva such as eczema or lichen sclerosis

However, some women may also need lubricants because they just don't produce enough secretions for no obvious reason. Anxiety can cause a reduction in natural vaginal lubrication; so try to relax and enjoy your intimate moments.

Some women think that an estrogen cream can be used as a lubricant but this is not true. You should apply your estrogen cream to the vulva once daily at the same time each day and many women apply it after their shower.

A lubricant is applied just before or during sex, if you feel you are becoming too dry in the vulva or vagina. Lots of different brands of lubricants are available at your local drugstore. Some products such as Vaseline or mineral based oils should not be used with condoms as they weaken the latex. The product called Replens is not a lubricant to be used during sex; it is a moisturizer used by women as an alternative to estrogen cream.

Some personal lubricants contain the antiseptic called chlorhexidine that can cause irritation and allergies and is toxic to sperm. So read the labels carefully. Some lubricants contain the preservative called propylene glycol which causes irritation in some women. Don't use too much of any lubricant as it will be messy.

I have found that natural oils work best; they are not chemical based and will not cause allergies or irritations. Good choices are castor oil, olive oil or coconut oil, which have lubricant and moisturizing effects and can soothe irritations. Organic cold pressed coconut oil has a fragrant but subtle tropical aroma.

Gels and creams to enhance the sensitivity

These gels contain the amino acid L-Arginine in variable amounts and I use a compounding pharmacist who uses a strength of 300mg per dose. This gel is applied to the clitoris at the beginning of sex. The L-Arginine acts as a vasodilator to increase the flow of blood to the clitoris.

6. Treatment of low sex drive

Stay young and sexy with bio-identical hormones

There are three different bio-identical sex hormones –

- Progesterone
- Estrogen
- Testosterone

Progesterone therapy

Progesterone is a sex hormone that is made by the ovaries during the latter half of the menstrual cycle and in vast amounts by the placenta during pregnancy. Progesterone exerts a calming effect and can promote emotional contentment and stability. The brain has receptors for progesterone and this is why natural hormones can be so beneficial for emotional disorders.

If you find that your mood and/or sex drive lowers during the one to two weeks before your menstrual bleeding commences, then you will probably benefit from natural progesterone.

Progesterone deficiency is very common in women today because they often delay pregnancy to later in life and have fewer pregnancies. Progesterone deficiency can cause unpleasant symptoms such as loss of sex drive, anxiety, irritability and depression. Progesterone deficiency can also cause physical health problems such as heavy and/or painful menstrual bleeding, endometriosis, fibroids, pelvic congestion, an increased risk of cancer, premenstrual headaches, polycystic ovarian syndrome and unexplained infertility.

The good news is that natural progesterone therapy can often alleviate these symptoms in women of all ages. Thus one would think that natural progesterone is commonly prescribed for these diverse and common problems. In reality few doctors prescribe natural progesterone because it cannot be patented by drug companies. Thus drug companies do not promote natural progesterone or educate doctors about its use or benefits. This is a pity and results in much unneeded suffering.

It must be Natural Progesterone

I recommend only the use of natural progesterone, which has a chemical structure identical to the progesterone produced by the ovaries. Natural progesterone is made in the laboratory from the plant hormone called diosgenin found in soybeans and sweet potatoes (yams). Because natural progesterone is identical to the progesterone produced by the ovaries it is called a *bio-identical hormone.*

Unfortunately, doctors often prescribe strong synthetic progesterones called 'progestogens', mistakenly believing that they will have the same effect as natural progesterone. This is not true and synthetic progesterone will usually make most of your symptoms worse and will not help your sex drive. Many of these synthetic progestogens are derived from male (testosterone-like) synthetic hormones and so may cause side effects such as increased appetite, depression, irritability, low libido, weight gain, fluid retention, acne, greasy skin and increased cholesterol. These synthetic progestogen hormones attach onto the natural progesterone receptors found throughout the body and brain, but they cannot switch on all these receptors. Only natural progesterone can turn on ALL the progesterone receptors just as a key turns and releases a lock. So you can understand that synthetic progestogens will not have the same beneficial effect as natural progesterone.

Natural progesterone is not as effective if taken by mouth (orally), as it is destroyed by the liver enzymes after its absorption from the intestines.

Therefore, natural progesterone is best administered by routes that bypass the liver such as –

- Creams – which may be rubbed into the skin (transdermal) or inserted high up into the vagina
- Vaginal pessaries or suppositories

Natural progesterone can also be given in the form of lozenges known as *troches*, which are NOT designed to be sucked or chewed or swallowed. Theoretically the troche is held between the upper gum and the cheek until it is completely absorbed, with the hormone it contains being transferred directly into the bloodstream across the mucous lining of the oral cavity.

Natural progesterone can also be administered in the form of capsules which contain tiny (micronized) particles of progesterone. Theoretically these tiny particles of progesterone are more resistant to breakdown by the enzymes in the gut and the liver, so that more progesterone gets into the bloodstream.

By giving natural progesterone in these ways, we are aiming to bypass the liver so that the progesterone can be absorbed directly into the circulation and carried to the progesterone receptors on your cells.

How to use Natural Progesterone

Generally, natural progesterone therapy is started five days after the end of your menstrual bleeding. The progesterone is then continued daily up to the first day of your menstrual bleeding. Once your bleeding starts the progesterone should be stopped. If you find it difficult to judge when to begin using the progesterone, you can start it at the time of ovulation, which is normally 14 days before the expected onset of your menstrual bleeding. Make sure you stop the progesterone on the first day of your menstrual bleeding and this way the progesterone is fitting in with your own natural cycle.

Each woman is an individual and trial and error using different dosages, forms and schedules of progesterone may be required before the symptoms are fully under control.

My personal preference is to administer natural progesterone in the form of a cream, which is rubbed into the skin of the inner upper arms or the inner upper thighs. You should apply the cream to dry skin after your shower, and if you shower or bathe twice daily, then it may be more effective to apply the cream twice daily after each shower. The cream needs to be rubbed very thoroughly into the skin so that the entire amount is well absorbed into the skin, with no cream remaining visible or detectable on the skin. The cream can be used once or twice daily and required doses vary. The average effective doses are 30mg to 100mg daily.

Some doctors are very cynical about the use of creams containing natural progesterone because they do not believe that the progesterone is effectively absorbed through the skin in to the bloodstream. In other words, they do not think that clinically effective amounts of progesterone can be achieved in the body by using the creams. However, a study published in the American Journal of Obstetrics & Gynecology in 1999 found that absorption of progesterone from creams was just as good as absorption of estrogen from patches. They concluded that the application of progesterone cream to the skin appeared to be a safe and effective route of administration. [13]

Progesterone Troches

Natural Progesterone troches are lozenges that are placed between the upper gum and the cheek. They slowly dissolve through the mucous membrane of the cheek and the progesterone is absorbed directly into the circulation. Do not suck, chew or swallow the lozenges. They come in a variety of flavors. Capsules containing micronized progesterone can be swallowed.

The average dose is 50mg daily but the dose may range from 25 to 200mg daily. It is given for the 14 days before menstrual bleeding.

The benefits of the progesterone troches are that they are convenient to carry around, and like the progesterone cream, they relieve the symptoms of premenstrual syndrome such as low libido, mood disorders, insomnia, pelvic congestion, migraines, heavy bleeding, menstrual pain and fatigue.

If doses are excessive, some breakthrough bleeding, drowsiness and fluid retention may occur. In some women, the troche may produce irritation of the gum. In allergy-prone people, the troches may cause allergic type symptoms such as rashes and swelling. The progesterone cream is best used in allergy-prone people. If the troches contain sugar they may increase dental caries. If these side effects occur then reduce the dosage of hormones in the troche, or change to the progesterone cream.

Notes on Natural Progesterone

Natural progesterone is not a contraceptive and indeed will increase fertility!

Natural progesterone does not work if you are taking the oral contraceptive pill.

In Australia, you will need a doctor's prescription for natural progesterone and it is made up into a cream by a compounding pharmacist. In the USA, a prescription is not needed although this may change.

See page 95 for contact details for compounding chemists.

For more information contact my Women's Health Advisory Service in the USA on 623 334 3232 or in Australia on 02 4655 8855 or email ehelp@liverdoctor.com

Side effects of Natural Progesterone Cream

Possible side effects include some breakthrough bleeding if doses are excessive. Breakthrough bleeding is more likely to occur if the cream is inserted high up in the vagina. When used vaginally, some vaginal irritation may occur if the base of the cream is unsuitable.

If the progesterone cream causes vaginal irritation, speak to your compounding pharmacist about changing the base of the cream. Alternatively, just use the cream on the skin of the inner upper arms or inner upper thighs.

Excessive doses of progesterone can lead to bloating and drowsiness. If you have any of the side effects, reduce the dose until the side effects disappear. As you can see the required dose can vary a lot, as every woman is an individual, and by experimenting with the dose of the cream, you can avoid any nuisance side effects.

Is Natural Progesterone safe?

Natural progesterone is very safe and is usually free of side effects. Pure natural progesterone does not cause birth defects or harm to the fetus if you become pregnant, and will reduce your chances of miscarriage. If you do fall pregnant whilst taking progesterone, continue to use it for the first 2 to 3 months of pregnancy. Notify your doctor if you are using progesterone once you fall pregnant.

Synthetic Progesterone

Synthetic progesterone (also known as progestogens) are available and common brand names are Norethisterone, Norgesterol, and Medroxy-progesterone acetate tablets. These tablets can be given every day, or for the 14 days before menstrual bleeding begins. The dosage varies depending upon the brand of tablet and the medical reason for which it is prescribed.

These synthetic progestogens have a slightly masculine effect, which may result in weight gain, pimples, greasy skin and hair. Some brands may cause fluid retention, moodiness, depression and elevation of cholesterol. They often make depression and other mood disorders much worse. They will not help your sex drive and may have the reverse effect, leading you to become more disinterested in sex!

Estrogen therapy

Natural estrogens may improve libido and sexual response and this is especially true in the following cases -

- Pre-menopausal and post-menopausal women
- After hysterectomy or after surgical sterilization with tubal clips; in these cases the ovaries may not work as well after surgery.

Estrogens improve the condition of the vagina and vulva and have the following effects –

- Strengthen and thicken the tissues making them more robust – thus you can tolerate longer sex or stronger sex
- Reduce dryness of the vagina and vulva
- Increase vaginal secretions

- Increase vaginal flexibility and stretchiness
- Improve bladder function and reduce bladder infections

Estrogen can increase the desire for sex and also makes the breasts and nipples more sensitive to touch. Estrogen keeps the breasts fuller and less droopy.

Types of Natural Estrogen

There are three types of natural estrogen produced by the ovaries and the fat tissue in your body; these are known as Estradiol, Estriol and Estrone.

If you need to take estrogen replacement therapy it is desirable to use bio-identical estrogens and not synthetic or animal derived estrogens such as Premarin. Bio-identical estrogens are synthesized in a laboratory from plant hormones – namely diosgenin in yams and stigmasterol in soy beans.

Bio-identical estrogens come in three different forms -

- Estradiol = E 2 is the strongest or most potent estrogen
- Estrone = E 1 is of medium strength
- Estriol = E 3 is the weakest estrogen of all the three estrogens

Estriol

Estriol is the safest of all forms of estrogen therapy. Even though estriol is not a potent estrogen, it has been proven to be effective for women with atrophic vaginitis. The symptoms of atrophic vaginitis include vaginal dryness, vaginal burning and irritation, vaginal itching and painful sexual intercourse.

Painful sexual intercourse is known as dyspareunia and is commonly caused by low estrogen levels. Generally speaking, after 4 weeks of treatment with estriol cream, the symptoms of atrophic vaginitis are relieved. Other good news is that estriol cream is free of side effects, except for an extremely rare possibility of allergy to the base used in the cream.

Estriol cream has also been found to be useful for preventing urinary tract infections in women with low estrogen levels. Estriol cream can

Increase your **Sex Drive** *naturally*

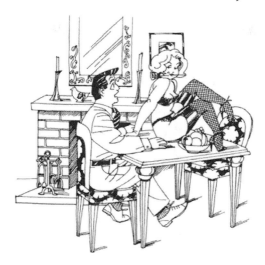

Women on natural hormones may start to behave in a more provocative way !

also greatly reduce urinary incontinence caused by weak pelvic floor muscles, laughing, coughing and straining. The estriol cream can be inserted into the vagina or rubbed on the vulva and the vaginal opening.

All three estrogens can be given in the form of creams, troches, tablets, gels or patches. These estrogens can be given singly or in combination; for example a product called Triest contains all three of the bio-identical estrogens and Biest contains estradiol and estriol.

Estrogens can be used cyclically for two to three weeks every month, or used every day. It is important to give some form of progesterone with the estrogen and I prefer natural progesterone, as it is more effective and safer.

The safest way to administer estrogen is in the form of creams or patches because the estrogen is absorbed through the skin into the bloodstream and does not go through the liver; thus we do not increase the risk of blood clots. If estrogen is given via the skin in creams or patches it will not increase the liver's production of Sex Hormone Binding Globulin (SHBG) – thus you will feel sexier!

Estrogen creams can be inserted into the vagina or used on the outside of the vaginal opening (around the vulva). Either way this prevents dryness and restores natural lubrication. Usually only small doses of estrogen are required and I most commonly use Estriol in a daily dose of 1mg to 2 mg. A doctor's script is required for all three types of estrogen.

Most doctors use branded estrogen creams such as Ovestin, which come with a vaginal applicator to insert the cream high up into the vagina. Ovestin contains the bio-identical estrogen called Estriol.

Other types of estrogen such as estrogen tablets or estrogen implants can be used, although they are relatively more potent and thus more likely to cause side effects such as tender breasts, migraines, leg cramps, fluid retention and an increased risk of blood clots.

The estrogen implants are relatively potent and may cause an increase in menstrual bleeding and other symptoms of estrogen dominance; thus they are best used only in women who have had a hysterectomy.

Since the results of the Women's Health Initiative Study were published in July 2002, all doctors have become aware that long term estrogen therapy will increase the risk of breast cancer. If the estrogen is combined with synthetic progesterone, this type of hormone therapy becomes even more risky to use long term, with an increased risk of blood clots and strokes. [17] Thus it is not wise to use potent forms of estrogen therapy for many years, and this means that estrogen implants are really only suitable for short term use. This means for not more than one year.

In my experience, I have found that estrogen implants can result in very high blood levels of estrogen being found on blood tests. This would be worrying if these women decided to continue with these potent forms of estrogen for many years. In contrast I have found that when using small doses of natural hormones in the form of creams, the blood levels of estrogen, progesterone and testosterone stay within safe and very modest levels.

I suggest that you stay with estrogen creams or patches, as the doses used can be much smaller and easily fine tuned to provide the smallest possible dose that relieves your symptoms and improves your sex life. I find that the creams are much easier to use than the patches because the creams can be applied to the vulva. The estrogen patches can cause skin irritations and do not always stick to the skin very well in hot and humid climates.

It is important to check the results of the estrogen therapy with regular blood or salivary estrogen levels, and suitable intervals are every 3 months initially and thereafter every 6 to 12 months.

Excessive doses or the more potent forms of estrogen are best avoided as they can lead to symptoms of estrogen dominance.

Estrogen dominance symptoms can include-

• Breast pain and lumpiness
• Fluid retention
• Gallstones
• Heavy or painful menstrual bleeding
• Increased size of fibroids
• Migraine headaches
• Aching legs and leg cramps
• Blood clots
• Weight gain in the hips and thighs

If these side effects occur you will need your doctor to reduce the dosage of estrogen, or change to the weakest form of estrogen which is estriol. I have found that small doses of an estriol only cream do not produce any side effects and this is my preferred treatment, especially for older women or for long term use.

Both natural progesterone and estrogens will reduce insomnia and hot flushes.

I usually prescribe a cream containing a combination of natural estrogen and progesterone. When it comes to the choice of which estrogen to use, I prefer to use estriol only or Biest estrogen, as it is weaker than Triest. A typical cream prescription for me to write would be Estriol 2.0mg and Progesterone 100mg per gram of cream, combined together in one cream with instructions to apply one gram daily to the vulva or the inner upper thigh. If you prefer, you can apply half a gram to the vulva and half a gram to the inner upper thigh. Rub in well after your shower.

I do not include the testosterone in the estrogen and progesterone cream because the dose of testosterone required to improve the sexual response will vary. I give the testosterone cream as a separate script and it is then easy for the patient to change the amount of testosterone cream if they get side effects.

Testosterone therapy

Testosterone is produced from cholesterol in the ovaries, adrenal glands and fat tissues. Testosterone is a powerful hormone in both sexes and when it comes to libido it can really be called the hormone of desire. It works to promote sexual desire in our brain and our genital organs and these areas of our body contain testosterone receptors. Testosterone receptors are found on the cells of the nipples, the clitoris and vagina.

Some women have very low levels of testosterone whilst others produce too much. Your level of testosterone is easily and accurately measured with a blood test. It is important to measure the levels of both total testosterone and free testosterone that are circulating in your blood. See page 92.

The test for total testosterone measures the absolute amount of testosterone in your blood including the amount that is bound to the protein Sex Hormone Binding Globulin (SHBG). SHBG acts like a transport vehicle to carry the testosterone around your bloodstream to the organs of the body that need it. When the testosterone is broken off the SHBG it becomes free and is thus able to act on your cells. It is only the free testosterone which is active on your cells and thus it is the type of testosterone that promotes libido.

The figures below show the amount of total testosterone in the blood that is considered normal.

Women
Total testosterone: 30 – 95ng/dL (nanograms per deciliter)

Men
Total testosterone: 300 to 1,200ng/dl (nanograms per deciliter)

If a male's testosterone levels drop below 500, their libido will reduce, often dramatically.

In women, you can see that the testosterone levels are much lower than in men and the normal range is much narrower.

This means that your body will be sensitive to relatively small changes in your blood testosterone level. For example, a reduction or an increase by 20ng/dl can make a big difference to your sexuality.

Low levels of testosterone can cause the following symptoms

- Low libido
- Reduced ability to orgasm
- A reduction in the size of your clitoris
- A reduction in the sensitivity of your clitoris
- A reduction in sexual fantasies
- Muscle aches and pains or muscle weakness
- Backache and chest wall pain
- Reduction of/or loss of pubic and armpit (axillary) hair

Low levels of testosterone can be caused by-

- Hysterectomy with removal of the ovaries – in some women, even if the ovaries are left in place during a hysterectomy (surgical removal of the uterus), we find that all the sex hormone levels drop to very low levels and never recover.
- Adrenal gland exhaustion or adrenal gland failure; thus it is important to have healthy adrenal gland function to supplement your body's production of testosterone.
- The oral contraceptive pill, which increases SHBG which binds the

testosterone.

- Postnatal depression.
- The pre-menopausal years when the ovaries are ageing and gradually producing less testosterone and other sex hormones.
- The post-menopausal years when the ovaries shrink and become inactive; although small amounts of testosterone continue to be produced from the ovaries even many years after menopause; but for many women it is nowhere near enough for them to feel sexually alive.

Very low levels of testosterone are more commonly seen in women with a low body weight and a low muscle mass. Your body type can influence the amount of testosterone that you produce.

Women who are overweight and carry most of their excess weight in the upper body and abdomen often have excess levels of testosterone and may have a higher libido because of this. This body shape is called the Android Body Shape or the apple shape. If an overweight, Android-shaped woman consumes high amounts of carbohydrate foods, especially sugar, this will lead to an increased production of testosterone. If an Android-shaped woman consumes more protein this will lead to lower levels of testosterone. Thus our diet can affect our hormones. To know your body shape do our interactive questionnaire at www.weightcontroldoctor.com and get your answer immediately.

How to use Testosterone

The best way to balance the testosterone levels in a woman is with a cream containing natural bio-identical testosterone. This testosterone is made in a laboratory using plant hormones such as diosgenin, as the starting material. Bio-identical hormones have the exact shape and structure as your own body's naturally produced hormones.

Bio-identical hormones have been popularized by the media and celebrities and I find that most women are aware that they are safer than synthetic hormones.

Previously, if a woman needed testosterone replacement she would usually be prescribed a synthetic form such as methyltestosterone in the form of tablets or injections. Methyltestosterone has a different chemical structure to the body's own naturally produced testosterone and is much stronger than bio-identical testosterone. Methyltestosterone was administered in tablet form and, because of this, was immediately processed by the liver after it was absorbed from the gut; thus the liver broke most of it down before it could get into the bloodstream. For this reason high doses of methyltestosterone were required and thus side effects such as masculinization and weight gain were more common. For these reasons many women were turned off using any male hormones to promote their sexual drive.

If we use testosterone creams, we can bypass the liver as the testosterone is absorbed via the skin into the blood circulation and is carried around the body to the cells that need it — all this happens before the liver can break it down.

This is much safer, as only very small doses of testosterone become effective this way. The low doses used in the cream are similar to the amounts of testosterone produced by your ovaries and adrenal glands and thus they do not produce big changes in your blood testosterone levels. We can easily adjust or *titrate* the dose of testosterone you need without any side effects being produced. One effect we do want to see however is a boost in your sex drive and sexual pleasure.

I find that the use of a cream containing testosterone allows the dose of testosterone to be easily measured and adjusted. For example, if we get the compounding pharmacy to make a testosterone cream containing 5mg of testosterone per gram of cream, we can measure amounts from 1/10th (.10) of a gram to 1 gram using a 1ml syringe or a 1 gram spoon. One gram is equivalent to a 1ml volume of the cream. If we started with 1 ml (1gram) of the cream we are getting 5 mg of testosterone and we can try this for several weeks to see if your libido improves. If you are worried about potential side effects start with 1/10th (.10) of a gram.

It is easy to adjust the dose down or up depending upon your response. The concentration of the testosterone in the cream can also be varied by the prescribing doctor and the compounding dispensing pharmacist so that you may want to try a lower strength cream of 1mg of testosterone per gram of cream for example.

I have found that the best place to apply the testosterone cream is on the vulva and make sure you get some on the clitoris. Some women just apply it to the clitoris and this works well for them. This is where the testosterone needs to work to keep your clitoris a normal size and to promote sensitivity of the clitoris and lips of the vulva. Your body will also absorb some of the testosterone from the vulva into the bloodstream, so this should increase your blood levels of testosterone into the normal healthy range.

After beginning testosterone cream, you should notice the difference within 2 weeks. The cream is used every day or every second day depending upon your preference and is rubbed into the clitoris and vulva. Apply the cream after your shower or last thing at night and rub it in well; you do not want to waste it, as it can be expensive. Do not apply just before sex or your partner will be getting some of your testosterone!

Bio-identical testosterone can be micronized and put in a capsule for swallowing. The term micronized means very fine particles which are theoretically better absorbed from a capsule. However the micronized testosterone, once absorbed from the gut, passes straight to the liver and the liver can easily break it down because it is a natural hormone.

Natural hormones are much easier for the liver to break down than synthetic hormones. I prefer to use testosterone creams and I generally do not prescribe testosterone capsules because of this liver effect.

Testosterone can be given in the form of troches, which are lozenges designed to be placed between the gum and the cheek. The troche needs to be kept in that position for around 20 minutes to allow the hormones to be absorbed across the mucus lining of the cheek directly into the blood circulation.

I don't prescribe troches very much because it is unavoidable that some of the hormones in the troche will be swallowed and thus go through the liver. This means that higher doses of hormones must be used in the troches compared to the creams. However, some women prefer the troches and find them effective.

Some women are very sensitive to testosterone and will get side effects if they use too much.

Side effects of excess testosterone include –

* Increase in facial hair
* Scalp hair loss especially in the frontal and temporal areas of the scalp
* Acne and pimples
* Increased aggression in mood and also in the bedroom! In this case your partner may come to see your doctor also asking for help to have his testosterone levels increased!

Some doctors do not understand the art and science of balancing a woman's hormones to make her feel *just right* when it comes to her sexuality. These doctors can be described as a *bull in a China shop*. This is one of the reasons that I have written this book because I have been doing this delicate juggling act for over 30 years. Many peri-menopausal and post-menopausal women struggle to restore their hormonal balance and libido because they are given the wrong doses and types of hormones.

For example, here is a typical scenario – a 50 year old woman has started menopause and her sex hormone levels have plummeted. This has caused loss of libido, vaginal dryness and fragility, hot flashes and insomnia and she decides that she needs hormone replacement therapy. Off she trots to her local doctor who does a blood test for menopause and proclaims to the patient, "Yes, you are menopausal and therefore you need estrogen!" This woman still has a uterus and thus she must be given progesterone along with the estrogen to protect her uterus from the increased risk of cancer incurred by taking estrogen alone. The patient is very happy to be given a tablet that contains estrogen combined with synthetic progesterone. Synthetic progesterone is called progestagen and has a different chemical structure to your own natural progesterone.

Initially the patient feels good, as her hot flashes are relieved and she can sleep. However, her libido is still zilch, gone and non-existent. Disappointed, the patient returns to the doctor complaining that she cannot stand the thought of sex and wants her sex drive back. The doctor responds by saying "Ah! You need more estrogen as this is the female hormone of desire". The doctor prescribes more estrogen but this does nothing, except cause fluid retention and migraines – what frustration for this poor woman!

The woman returns to the doctor several months later and says "I am over this, I am feeling awful and irritable; you must do something!" The doctor is way out of his depth (chances are he is male, but some female doctors do not understand hormones either!) The doctor prescribes anti-depressant drugs to ease this woman's negative moods and this is like adding fuel to the fire. Why? Because anti-depressants will further reduce her ability to achieve orgasm. This poor lady is not depressed; she has hormonal chaos created in her body from the combination of menopause and the wrong type of HRT.

The reason that the hormone tablets prescribed to this woman made her worse is that they were absorbed straight into the liver and this caused the liver to start making extra amounts of the binding protein called SHBG. The SHBG started to bind and inactivate the prescribed hormones she was taking as well as her own testosterone. This caused her free testosterone levels to drop and she started to feel more and more turned off sex. Her doctor did not realize that this could be overcome by ceasing the oral hormones and replacing them with hormones in a cream so that they bypassed the liver.

I see this scenario quite a lot and really I can feel sorry for the doctors and the patients because, without the understanding of bio-identical hormones, these doctors are lost at sea and way out of their depth.

They must feel helpless when confronted by a woman who is a hormonal mess and wants her libido back — or else! This is why you must educate yourself so you can let the doctor know what you require or else seek the services of a doctor who specializes in bio-identical sex hormones.

Just as women need to be assertive in the bedroom, they need to be assertive with their doctors and you can do it in a non confrontational way and even suggest to the doctor what you would like in your cream.

Some women take the hormone DHEA (spelt dehydroepiandrosterone) because they think it works the same as testosterone. They also think that it can get turned into testosterone and estrogen in their ovaries. This is not true, as once your ovaries have stopped making hormones they cannot use any raw material type hormones.

DHEA acts in your body like a weaker form of testosterone but it does not have the libido enhancing effects of real testosterone. I use DHEA in women with poor adrenal gland function and chronic fatigue and it is helpful for these problems.

I have had patients addicted to testosterone because it makes them feel like a superwoman! One particular patient, who is in her 50s, gets her local doctor to give her testosterone injections every month and these injections contain a high dose. She does have some extra facial and body hair and a slightly deep voice but she does not care! If she does not get her testosterone shots, she feels 200 years old and has awful fatigue, depression and muscle and bone pain. She does not use testosterone primarily for sex drive but she uses it for her wellbeing.

Another patient of mine had suffered with a chronic back ache and chest wall pain for 20 years. After 6 weeks on testosterone replacement she was pain free and no longer needed to take pain killers. Wow, that's impressive!

Apart from its sexual enhancing effects, testosterone has other positive effects and can –

- Boost energy
- Reduce depression
- Reduce muscle and bone pain
- Increase bone density
- Increase muscle bulk and muscle strength
- But we do not want to overdose on testosterone or we may change from superwoman into superman!

Is Testosterone safe?

Generally speaking, low doses of bio-identical testosterone are very safe. This is logical, as we are only using doses that keep the blood levels of testosterone in the normal or physiological range.

This is what your own ovaries and adrenal glands would do, if they were working properly. With age, however, their hormonal output diminishes and we begin to suffer the symptoms of testosterone deficiency. Oral synthetic testosterone is not as safe as the low doses of natural testosterone used in the creams. Large doses or synthetic testosterone may cause an increase in cholesterol levels.

If you take long term hormones you need your regular blood checks of cholesterol levels and liver function in addition to checking your levels of testosterone and other hormones. If the testosterone level is too high, we simply reduce the dose, which is really easy to do with a cream.

You will not become masculinized if small doses of testosterone are used. There are few long term studies on the use of testosterone but I think it is very safe and I have never seen it cause any serious side effects or cancer.

Sex after cancer

Many women suffer with severe sexual dysfunction after treatment for breast cancer or other hormone sensitive cancers.

Cancers that are sensitive to the growth stimulating effects of estrogen are breast and uterine cancers and, to a lesser degree, ovarian cancers. Treatment for breast, ovarian and uterine cancer results in extremely low levels of estrogen and progesterone. The very commonly prescribed drugs called aromatase inhibitors used in post menopausal breast cancer patients, work by blocking the production of estrogen in the fat tissues; this results in extremely low levels of estrogen in the blood and in the tissues of the vaginal and vulva.

Without help, sex will become unpleasant and difficult.

The use of oral hormone replacement therapy to relieve symptoms of estrogen deficiency after breast cancer is generally not recommended.

A Swedish study reported in the journal, The Lancet, found that breast cancer survivors who took oral hormone replacement therapy had over three times as many breast cancer recurrences as survivors who did not take any HRT. [1]

This is not surprising as the Women's Health Initiative (WHI) study testing oral estrogens and synthetic progestagens in healthy post menopausal women was stopped early in July 2002 because the researchers found that the hormones caused an increased risk of breast cancer, clots and heart disease. [17]

There is limited research on the risks of HRT in women who have had other types of cancer such as ovarian and uterine cancer.

So what can women with hormone sensitive cancers do if their sex life is in tatters due to non-existent levels of estrogen and progesterone?

Well, the safest thing to do is to avoid all oral forms of estrogen and progesterone (including bio-identical types and including troches).

Oral estrogens and progestagens are the types of hormones proven to increase the risk of breast cancer and breast cancer recurrences. This, however, does not mean we cannot safely use other ways of delivering hormones to local tissues where they are needed.

The safest way to use bio-identical hormones is in the form of creams in very small doses. It is even safer if you only apply the cream to the vulva and the opening of the vagina; in other words do not put the cream high up into the vagina. There are no long term studies of the effects of estrogen and progesterone creams applied to the vulva in survivors of breast cancer and other types of hormone sensitive cancers; however if used in small doses, I believe the creams are safe.

If you have had breast cancer or uterine cancer, it is not wise to use the forms of estrogen called estradiol or estrone, as these are more potent and can stimulate receptors on breast and uterine tissue. The safest estrogen to use is estriol. Estriol is water soluble and does not build up in the body and is not a potent estrogen; for these reasons it is much safer. I also think it is desirable and safe to include some natural progesterone in the cream because progesterone is thought to have anti-cancer effects. [10]

We have learnt that natural testosterone is a potent libido enhancer for women and if your blood testosterone levels are very low, a small amount of testosterone in a cream can be applied to the vulva and clitoris; this will not increase the risk of cancer recurrence, as we are using only small doses, and it is only having a local effect on the vulva where it is needed.

If I had a breast cancer survivor patient with a very dry and painful vagina who is consequently unable to enjoy any sexual activity I would prescribe the following:

Cream One: Estriol 1.5mg and progesterone 30mg per gram of cream; apply half to one gram daily to the vulva and clitoris

Cream Two: Testosterone 2mg per gram of cream; apply half to one gram daily to vulva and clitoris

These are low doses and can be easily adjusted up and down by varying the amount of cream. Doses can be checked with blood tests every three to six months.

Oxytocin – the love and cuddle hormone

Oxytocin is a natural hormone produced in the hypothalamus and pituitary gland.

Synthetic oxytocin has been used for decades to induce or speed up uterine contractions during childbirth and is given intravenously for this purpose. Oxytocin is required for breast feeding as it acts on the mammary glands to excrete milk into the nipples.

Oxytocin requires magnesium to work on its receptors; thus if you are magnesium deficient, oxytocin does not work effectively in your body.

Several studies have shown that blood levels of oxytocin increase during orgasm in both sexes. [5, 6, 7]

Brain

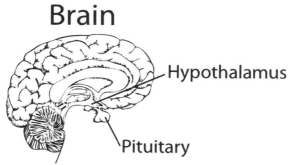

Studies confirm that oxytocin plays an important role in sexual stimulation and arousal. Oxytocin promotes human bonding and trust which is required for romance and emotional attachment between couples. Oxytocin may inhibit the parts of the brain (such as the amygdyla) that make us fearful, conservative and over controlled and this effect may be very helpful for women who become anxious about having sex. Because of these relaxing and calming effects, oxytocin helps us to let go, which increases the chances of having an orgasm.

Blood levels of oxytocin have been found to be increased by self stimulated orgasm (during masturbation) and stimulation of the nipples, vulva and vagina.

Oxytocin nasal sprays are available on prescription where a precise dosage can be controlled and absorption is good through the nasal mucous membranes.

Oxytocin body sprays are ineffective because of poor absorption. Oxytocin tablets are ineffective because the oxytocin is quickly destroyed by the digestive enzymes in the gut and thus does not get into the bloodstream. Some doctors prescribe oxytocin lozenges (troches) with 50 units per troche and this is designed to be placed in-between the gum and the cheek for absorption across the oral mucous membrane. The sexual arousal effect is said to last for at least one day, but these are anecdotal stories.

Generally speaking, oxytocin therapy is safe and side effects are not common; the most common side effect from the nasal spray is a mild headache which passes when the oxytocin wears off. Allergic reactions are possible in those who are allergy prone.

Oxytocin is unstable and is destroyed by heat and light so you need to keep it refrigerated or carry it in an ice pack.

The use of oxytocin nasal spray as a love and orgasm enhancer is relatively new and is an off label usage still considered experimental. Oxytocin nasal spray is generally prescribed by doctors to improve lactation in nursing mothers. Oxytocin nasal sprays have been studied in patients with social phobias, social anxiety, autism and schizophrenia with encouraging results. Thus oxytocin may not only help to stimulate erotic pleasures, it may also reduce anxiety in those who fear sex. It may also help those with post traumatic stress disorder.

Not all pharmacies can supply oxytocin nasal spray. The University of Washington Medical Center Pharmacy provides oxytocin nasal spray bottles in a concentration of 10 units/ml. Stronger doses (20 to 50 units/ml) according to your doctor's prescription, can be made up by a compounding pharmacist. Start with a low concentration and use 1 spray in each nostril and work with your doctor to find the dose that ignites your passion.

If you don't like the feeling of spray up your nose, you can tilt your head backwards and drip the oxytocin liquid into each nostril; one spray = one drop. Some people prefer to spray under their tongue or the back of their throat but this will not produce as good absorption as the nasal route of delivery.

Female Viagra – Does it work?

Since the release of Viagra in 1998, the sex life of men has been revo-lutionized, however for women, the subject of their sexuality extends beyond the aspect of physical performance.

Viagra has been studied in thousands of women and has been found to have variable and only modest effects. A female form of Viagra called Tadalafil is branded for use by women as Ladialis.

Tadalafil does not increase sexual desire in women and it has no effect upon their hormones. Despite this, some women find it of benefit.

A study carried out by Dr Jennifer Berman at the University of California compared women on placebo to women on Viagra. The study included women aged from 30 to 71 who were either post menopausal or who had a hysterectomy. The study looked at two things-

• If there were differences in the sensation in the vagina, labia or clitoris during intercourse or stimulation of the vulva.

• If there were differences in pleasure and satisfaction during foreplay and intercourse.

Viagra was found to be more useful in women with Female Sexual Arousal Disorder (FSAD). FSAD is defined as the inability to progress through the normal stages of sexual arousal and is often associated with physical problems such as reduced blood flow to the vulva and lack of vaginal lubrication.

This is in contrast to women who suffer with Hypoactive Sexual Desire Disorder (HSDD) characterized by lack of interest in sex or aversion to sex; in HSDD the effects of Viagra or Tadalafil are minimal and really do not help. In women with lack of interest (HSDD), the use of hormones and oxytocin are likely to be of much more benefit.

An eight year study by the drug company Pfizer, with 3,000 women, showed that Viagra had a limited benefit in women with sexual dysfunction – the reason they said was that men and women have a different relationship between arousal and desire.

For men, arousal almost always leads to desire for sex but in women, arousal and desire are often not connected. The researchers concluded that it is not the genital organs but the brain that is the most crucial organ in women when it comes to being turned on. Although Viagra caused increased flow of blood to the pelvic area, women under this effect were not found to feel any increase in sexual arousal.

The main benefits of Viagra were in women on anti-depressant drugs and the researchers found that Viagra reduced the sexual dysfunction side effects caused by anti-depressant drugs in around two-thirds of the women studied. In the women taking anti-depressant drugs, the action of Viagra to increase blood flow to the genital organs helped increase sexual arousal and lubrication. The Pfizer researchers found that Viagra could be helpful in some women who had once had normal sex drive but then suddenly lost all sexual desire. Women who had always had a problem with low sex drive were not helped by Viagra.

Tadalafil and Viagra are taken as tablets and start to work 45 minutes after taking the tablet; their effects lasts 12 to 24 hours.

Possible side effects of Viagra or Tadalafil include:

A slight increase in heartbeat rate and a slight decrease in blood pressure. Some women experience a slight headache and dizziness. Do not take Tadalafil or Viagra if you are having more than one alcoholic drink or taking recreational drugs known as poppers (such as amyl nitrate or butyl nitrate).

If you have heart problems, your doctor may not prescribe Viagra or Tadalafil.

7. Strategies to strengthen your immune system

These strategies will improve the health of the tissues of the vagina and vulva making them less prone to inflammation. You will also find that you will get fewer infections of the vagina and bladder, if you are prone to these. In fact, you will find that your whole body will become healthier, not just your genital areas.

If you suffer with genital herpes your attacks will become less frequent and less severe. Unpleasant discharge and odor, due to bacterial infections of the vagina, will be controlled and gradually disappear. You will have less candida or thrush. If you suffer with chronic inflammatory disorders of the vulva (such as Lichen Sclerosis or dermatitis etc.), these strategies are essential, as they treat the cause of these problems.

Chronic infection of the vulva, vagina and/or cervix with the Human Papilloma Virus (HPV) can also be controlled using these strategies. The HPV can only cause symptoms or disease if your immune system is weak. By strengthening the immune system with nutritional medicine the HPV will not be able to damage your genital areas. Thus recurrent and unsightly warts of the vulva, which are caused by the HPV, will disappear although this may take 3 to 6 months.

This program will help to reduce vulvodynia, and indeed often cures it, as it is reducing the inflammation in the nerves and tissues of the vulva. The only extra thing to consider with vulvodynia is that you will need a magnesium supplement.

This program will also improve the circulation of blood to your genital areas.

These strategies need to be followed long term because there is always a need to optimize our immune function. Results may take anywhere from 6 weeks to 12 months, so you need to be persistent and regular with the supplements and dietary improvements.

Here are the essential strategies:

- Take a selenium supplement in a dose of 200mcg daily; use the selenomethionine form of selenium as it is organic and readily available from drug stores or health food stores. Selenium exerts many benefits in your immune system and is essential to overcome recurrent viral infections, such as genital herpes and the Human Papilloma Virus (HPV). Selenium is also anti-inflammatory and thus reduces inflammatory conditions of the vulva such as dermatitis and Lichen Sclerosis. Selenium has proven cancer preventative properties so you don't want to be low in this mineral. [8]

- Take a zinc supplement in a dose of 10mg to 20mg daily, as this will reduce infections such as candida, herpes and HPV. Zinc is also important to control inflammation.

- Boost your intake of omega 3 fatty acids by taking fish oil and/or by consuming walnuts, chia seeds and flaxseeds on a regular basis. I take 1 to 2 dessertspoons of fish oil every day to reduce inflammation. Keep your fish oil in the fridge and take it just before you eat your meal.

  Purchase some whole flaxseeds and grind them into a powder using a coffee grinder or food processor. You may store the flaxseed powder in the freezer or grind it freshly daily. I recommend you consume 1 to 2 tablespoons daily. This is a great way to keep your bowels regular as well.

  The omega 3 fatty acids will overcome many painful and/or irritating disorders of the vulva such as dermatitis, eczema and Lichen Sclerosis. The omega 3 fatty acids will also reduce dryness of the vulva and vagina and reduce your susceptibility to genital infections.

- Increase the quantity of healthy bacteria in your intestines and vagina by consuming plain unflavored full fat Greek style yogurt regularly — ideally every day. If you don't like the tart taste of Greek yogurt, add fresh fruit and ground flaxseed to the yogurt.

You can also take a good quality probiotic supplement containing healthy bacteria to improve the health of your intestines and vagina. These strategies are essential if you have bacterial vaginosis or candida.

• Ensure that you are not deficient in vitamin D. Vitamin D acts like an anti-inflammatory hormone in your body and increases immune strength. Vitamin D deficiency is a huge problem and is widespread. There is an increasing amount of evidence to show a link between low levels of vitamin D and the inability of your immune system to fight off a viral illness. Vitamin D supplementation has been associated with improved outcomes for osteoporosis, immune disorders and cancer.

In addition to skin manufacture from sunlight, vitamin D can be found in such foods as oily fish, canned fish, cod liver oil, liver, eggs, dairy products and fortified juice. It is also available in supplement form, with the current recommendation being that you take between 400 and 1000 IU of vitamin D 3 daily. Many people, especially those who avoid the sun or those living in cold countries, need much more than this and doses of around 5000 IU daily may be needed before you can get your blood levels of vitamin D into the higher desirable range.

It is easy to check your body's levels of vitamin D with a simple blood test; if your levels are below or at the lower limit of the normal range please take a vitamin D 3 supplement and/or get some sunshine on your skin. Recheck your blood levels after 3 months to ensure your vitamin D increases to the higher limit of the normal range. Make sure that you do not become deficient in vitamin D again.

Ask your doctor to check your blood level of vitamin D. Vitamin D can be measured in two different units of measurement and in the USA the units used are ng/mL. In Australia and Canada, the units of measurement are nmol/L. The normal ranges of vitamin D by different laboratories can vary significantly and you will be surprised by the large range between lower normal and upper normal – see table over the page.

Lower Limit Vitamin D in blood	Upper Limit Vitamin D in blood
75 nmol/L	*200 nmol/L*
30 ng/mL	*80 ng/mL*

You don't want to be average here; you want to have levels of vitamin D that optimize your immune system to fight infection and inflammation. The optimal levels of vitamin D are higher than the average levels.

I recommend you take enough supplements of vitamin D 3 and/or get enough sunshine to keep your serum vitamin D levels around 150 to 200 nmol/L or 70 to 80ng/mL. Vitamin D 3 supplements are not expensive and are widely available and should be taken with food.

Excess vitamin D intake can cause elevated blood calcium levels; so don't overdose on it - it's not a case of the more the better. Get your blood level checked every 6 months to find the dose of vitamin D 3 that keeps you in the optimal levels.

- Ensure that you are not deficient in iodine, as this mineral is essential for thyroid function. If your thyroid is sluggish, this will reduce your production of progesterone — an important hormone for emotional and physical sexual relationships.

Iodine acts as a natural antibiotic; if you are low in iodine your immune system will be weakened and you will be more prone to vaginal and skin infections. Check your iodine levels and if your result shows a deficiency, take an iodine supplement. I recommend that you take an iodine supplement anyway because it is so important for immune health and energy levels. One billion people are at risk of severe iodine deficiency. I have found that around 50% of my patients in Australia are deficient in iodine. The best way to test your body's level of iodine is with a urine test which measures the concentration of iodine in your urine.

I have formulated an excellent product called *Thyroid Health Capsules* and each capsule contains Selenomethionine 100mcg, Iodine 162mcg and Vitamin D 3 1000 units.

Iodine status of patient	Urinary iodine concentration
Severe iodine deficiency	*Less than 20 mcg/Liter*
Moderate iodine deficiency	*20 to 49 mcg/Liter*
Mild iodine deficiency	*50 to 99 mcg/Liter*
Not iodine deficient	*Over 100 mcg/Liter*

- Avoid consuming excess sugar as sugar feeds infections and promotes inflammation. This all adds up to more candida and more unhealthy vaginal bacteria. Many women find that by avoiding refined sugars they are able to control unpleasant vaginal odor. Instead of sugar, eat fresh fruits and plain yogurt.

- If you have bowel problems such as constipation, hemorrhoids, flatulence or irritable bowel syndrome this can be a real turn off for sex. In such cases a probiotic supplement and Greek yogurt will really help a lot. Drink more water, take a gluten free fiber supplement such as Fibertone powder and a ground flaxseed powder. If you have a chronic skin problem (such as dermatitis or Lichen Sclerosis etc.) in the vulva area and/or around the anus, try avoiding gluten containing foods.

- Increase the amount of raw fruits and vegetables in your diet and aim for at least 30% of your diet to consist of raw foods. Good choices of raw foods include fruit, vegetable salads, raw nuts and seeds and sprouted legumes and seeds.

- Raw juicing can also help a lot to reduce inflammation and increase immune and gut health. Raw juices have the ability to reduce your risk of cancer and to help you overcome and cure cancer. A juice machine is a worthwhile investment! Good things to juice are citrus, cabbage, kale, beet, carrot, apple, ginger, celery and fresh green herbs such as mint, parsley and cilantro. If you are super busy, you can make a week's supply of juice and freeze it in glass jars. If you freeze it immediately after making it, the healing properties will be retained. You will find benefit from drinking 7 to 8 ounces (200 to 300mls) of juice daily. I like to drink my juice whist it is defrosting and it gives the experience of having a *slushy* but this time it's a healthy one!

- Use natural antibiotics. If you suffer with recurrent infections, you may become a victim of the overuse and dependence on antibiotic drugs. These drugs will destroy the good bacteria in your gut and vagina and eventually lead to more infections. By strengthening your immune system you will get far fewer infections. You can also use natural antibiotics such as vitamin C, garlic, onions and radishes of all varieties, cloves, thyme and olive leaf extract. You can purchase them as capsules, liquids or include them in your juices and diet.

- Colloidal silver can help to fight bacterial infections and some women get good results by taking a course of this every six months; the dose is generally one teaspoon daily in water or juice. One teaspoon of colloidal silver can be added to your tea tree vaginal douche gel solution and helps to overcome bacterial and yeast infections of the vagina.

- By consuming small amounts of natural antibiotics on a regular basis your immune system will improve in leaps and bounds!

8. Natural supplements to improve your sex drive and performance

A wide range of natural products are available to enhance both male and female sexual enjoyment. Many of these products are herbs which have been used traditionally to increase genital blood flow. Generally speaking, these herbs are safe, although you should check with your doctor if you are taking prescriptions medications, as herbs can interact with some of these. You must be cautious with the herb yohimbine, which can have side effects if you use too much.

Natural products such as herbs can only have a mild or subtle effect on sex drive and/or performance and they cannot produce the same effects as Viagra, prescription sex hormones or oxytocin. Femme-Phase is an excellent formulation, which contains a mixture of phyto-estrogens from herbs and foods and is designed to balance sex hormones during the pre-menstrual and peri-menopausal phases of a woman's life. Many women find FemmePhase helpful for their libido as well as their general health.

Each FemmePhase capsule contains:

The herbs Black Cohosh, Dong Quai, Licorice, Sage, Sarsaparilla, Rosehips, Wild Yam, Horsetail and Kelp. Vitamin C, Bioflavonoids, Vitamin D, Vitamin E, four different types of Calcium, Magnesium, Zinc, Folic Acid, Vitamin K, Vitamins B1, B2 and B6.

These are some of the many herbs that are sold in drugstores or online to enhance sexual performance and enjoyment:

- Wild yam
- Rhodiola
- Ginseng
- Fo-ti
- Longjack root
- Pygeum africanum

- Sarsaparilla
- Ginger extract
- Ganoderma lucidum
- Cordyceps sinensis
- Tribulus terrestris
- Coleus forskohlii
- Damiana
- Mucuna pruriens
- Muira puama
- Passion flower
- Rehmannia
- Smilax myosotiflora
- Polyrachis vicinia
- Tongkat Ali (a Malaysian herb)
- Horny goat weed
- Ginkgo Biloba
- Ashwagandha (Indian ginseng and Ayurvedic ginseng)
- Maca root (Peruvian ginseng)
- Yohimbine from African yohimbine tree bark is a controversial herb and some insurance companies do not insure manufacturers of this product. Yohimbine stimulates blood flow to the genital organs. If you use too much it can cause nausea, dizziness, anxiety, a drop in blood pressure and abdominal pain.

If you decide to use herbs for your sex life, it is not a case of *the more the better*. You may get side effects if you take too much, so stick to the recommended dose on the label.

If the natural herbs do not work for you this is a sign that you should see your doctor for hormone or oxytocin treatment or at least a proper diagnosis. *For more information contact my Women's Health Advisory Service in the USA on 623 334 3232 or in Australia on 02 4655 8855 or email ehelp@liverdoctor.com*

9. Foods to increase your sex drive

Chocolate

The best known food to put you and your partner in the mood is chocolate. One variation is chocolate body creams designed to be licked off by your partner. Chocolate contains phenylethylamine, which is thought to reproduce the emotional feeling of being in love. No wonder frustrated lovers often become chocoholics!

Eggs

Eggs are a wonderful food to boost your libido because they contain natural cholesterol and that's what your body makes sex hormones from. They are high in protein and sulfur and that's good for your liver — you need a healthy liver to have healthy hormone levels. Eggs are low in carbohydrate so they will not cause weight gain. Choose free range organic eggs if possible.

Oysters

Of course we have all heard about oysters as the classic aphrodisiac! Oysters are high in dopamine which is the chemical that makes us feel pleasure and satisfaction. Oysters are a good source of zinc which is needed for testosterone production. If you don't like the taste of oysters, substitute anchovies or mussels instead.

Bananas

Bananas are not only the classic phallic symbol they are also good for your libido because they are high in potassium which is needed for muscular energy.

Seeds and nuts

Walnuts, chia seeds and flaxseeds are high in essential fatty acids of the omega 3 variety. The omega 3 fats elevate mood and increase the health of your vagina and vulva.

Avocado

Avocado is a delicious and non fattening healthful treat that was called *the testicle tree* by the Aztecs. Avocados are very high in vitamin E which is essential for production of sex hormones and healthy blood vessels.

Green stuff

Green leafy vegetables and herbs (such as basil, mint, parsley, cilantro etc) are high in magnesium. It's a must to keep your magnesium levels at the high end of normal if you want to have a great sex life.

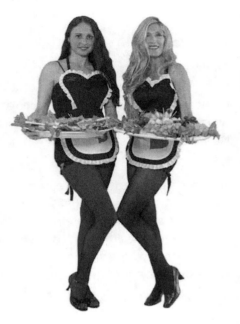

Magnesium is a superb enhancer of sexual function and energy because it relaxes the nervous system and opens up the arteries to optimize blood flow to the whole body, including the genital organs. It can help many women and men with erectile dysfunction and poor circulation.

You can also take a daily supplement of magnesium.

Exercise

Regular exercise is important and desirable and will improve the circulation of blood to all your vital organs, not just your pelvic organs and genitals. If you have arthritis or a back problem, the best exercise may be an indoor exercise bike and swimming. If you have lower back problems and a weakness of your spine, you probably have low core body strength. Start doing yoga or Pilates to build your core body strength and to improve abdominal and pelvic floor muscle strength.

Lower back problems can play havoc with your sex life. I had a male patient who had arthritis and disc bulging in his lower spine consequent to a workplace injury. This had made him completely impotent. No doctor could help him so he decided to help himself with an inversion table, which applies traction to the spinal vertebrae. After one week of using his inversion table he was fully functional again with normal erections. The traction had stopped the compression on his spinal cord and nerves and allowed the flow of blood and electrical energy to resume to his genitals. The same principle applies to women. You can see a good osteopath or chiropractor and also look into buying an inversion table. Inversion tables are not expensive and are easily purchased online

An analysis of 31,742 men aged 53 to 90 reported in the *Annals of Internal Medicine* in 2003 proved that exercise keeps you leaner and fit for sex, as well as mentally more ready for sexual interaction. The same applies to women.

10. Getting in the mood

The physical environment can be important for some people to put their mind on sex. Here are some creative and naughty tips!

Burn a candle or two (I have been told that red is the sexy color for candles) and you can burn an aromatic candle that makes the room smell sensual. Wear a nice perfume to enhance the sensual pleasure of love making. The sense of smell is located in the temporal lobes of the brain, close to the emotional and memory centers of the brain. Thus if you have great sex, the smell of your perfume will be remembered and this can put your partner in the mood next time he/she smells you.

Soft music, with a theme of love, can make lovemaking more romantic. Sexy lingerie can be a good turn on, especially if your partner takes it off really slow.

Many couples use sex toys to enhance their foreplay, but make sure you are not rough with them, as injuries can occur.

Massage oils can be very pleasant but it can be hard to get a man to give you a long sensual massage! Arousal gels containing L- arginine are available and you can ask your partner to rub your clitoris gently with this in a teasing way.

If you find it hard to relax, and this is common in a new relationship, you can have a cocktail – see my sister's cocktail recipe "Midnight Passion" to put you in the mood for love.

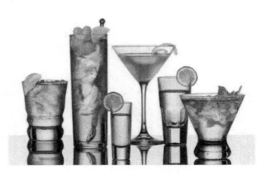

Midnight Passion

You will need a cocktail glass and your cocktail shaker filled with ice.

Ingredients:

2 ripe passion fruit pulps
6-8 drops liquid stevia
2 drops blue food coloring, or 6 blueberries
Juice of ½ lime
½ cup unsweetened banana and passion fruit juice, or plain passion fruit juice, or any other combination that you may fancy
1 sprig mint
A generous 3 count pour, or three second pour (it's the same thing) of vodka.

If using the blueberries, you will have to muddle them in the bottom of the shaker with your muddler before proceeding.

Fill the shaker three quarters full with ice and then add all other ingredients, including the mint. Shake vigorously and for at least one minute.

Pour into cocktail glass, garnish with small mint sprig.

This recipe is taken from my sister Madeleine's book, *The Low Carb Cocktail Party.* In her hey day, she was an erotic dancer, so she knows her stuff!

Often, a sensual movie can start the hormonal spark.

Sexual drive may diminish because of stress and a preoccupation with work. If you want to boost your sex life, start thinking about creative ways to make your relationship more exciting, erotic, romantic and more fun. Begin your day with that end in mind. If you want to make your sexual encounters wonderful for both of you, you can build your partner's confidence that he/she is attractive, sexy and the most important person in your life. You must feel sexy before you can be sexy. Use mischievous glances, smiles or a few carefully chosen words to create the reaction you want.

Your partner likes to know you care about their physical and mental wellbeing. That sets the scene for physical touches, massages and kisses that lead to sexual enjoyment for couples.

An excerpt from the memoirs of a *Red Hot Mama*

The following words are an excerpt from the memoirs of a *red hot mama* who spent thirty years as a counsellor.

Love and marriage go together like a horse and carriage, so says the old song of yesteryear. But what about love and sex? It should follow the same tune, and much of the time it does. So how do we achieve an exciting and fulfilling sex life instead of it becoming an elusive dream? If you follow a few old fashioned rules it can be quite simple – believe me!

Number one – and the most important – don't get too serious and remember to lighten up and enjoy your sex life. Being too serious about sex becomes stressful, fraught with insecurities and worries about your performance etc. Do not tread this perilous path! Always have that wonderful air of expectation – it is magnetic. Don't be concerned with imagined inadequacies or imperfections – just think about SEX!

I have lost count of the number of women of all ages and from all walks of life, who have asked me "What can I do about my flagging sex drive?" They often tell me quite openly that they have completely lost all sex drive and what is quite amazing is that they have husbands and partners who are loving and sexy men. I tell them they have got it made!

I am talking about everyday women in their thirties, forties and fifties, and some much older, who do not have life threatening issues or illness, some single, married, divorced who seemingly for no apparent reason have lost their sexual urge. After listening to their long and unhappy stories with commiseration, I always ask the question "Well what do you consider to be the greatest aphrodisiac?" This is always followed by a very long and pregnant pause, followed with a variety of interesting answers, but not one woman has ever verbalized the simple truth; this is that the greatest aphrodisiac is YOUR MIND.

When I tell them this simple truth it is usually met with absolute silence and sometimes disbelief. How often the obvious truth eludes us! Our subconscious mind governs our innermost feelings and desires. Your thoughts are your destination – so let's aim for the bedroom!

Before we go any further, let me tell you a funny story. One of my hilarious friends, around the age of fifty, confided that after being married for 25 years found her libido was severely flagging. To try and rekindle her libido she bought one of Jackie Collin's hot romance books. Well, she could not put the book down and every time her husband passed by the bedroom door, out would go her arm and drag him in. It worked a treat for their sex life and he considered it to be the best book in the house.

Get the chemistry of desire going and lift your spirits by getting in a positive confident state of mind and make a plan –

Purchase some sexy books or DVDs. Jackie Collins or Erica Jung write novels so hot the pages sizzle. It's all about sex and stirring your passion – wow, get ready to become a femme fatale! Start thinking romantic thoughts about your lover. Dwell upon the good sex you have had in the past and ways to improve on it even more. Be adventurous and creative in your plans. Be intimate – give him that telltale look and be generous with your kisses and cuddles.

Practise seduction with sexy body language, touching and being close. Leave love notes on his pillow or tuck them into his socks. Go for sexy underwear. If you are overweight, lose the excess pounds by exercising and eating fewer carbohydrates. This will make you more energetic and you will feel better about yourself.

Wear sexy clothes and jewelry and sing around the house or play romantic music – be cheerful!

Throw away your inhibitions and talk to your lover about what turns you on. Remember it is simple – it's all in the mind!

11. Sex therapy

Before 1966, sex therapy was considered a very murky and unscientific area. The publication of the bestselling book, *Human Sexual Response,* written by Masters and Johnson, was followed in 1970 by the opening of a clinic in St. Louis for sexual problems. The first generation of professional American sex therapists were created.

In the 1960s, sex was still often considered a taboo subject and masturbation was considered a bad habit and unhealthy by many cultures. Millions of women remained sexually and emotionally frustrated and developed physical symptoms because of this; these symptoms were usually treated with sedatives, pain killers or even smoking cigarettes!

Back in the days of the famous and brilliant (albeit controversial) Austrian psychiatrist, Sigmund Freud, the physical symptoms of women's emotional frustrations were called *hysterical*. Freud recognized that these physical symptoms were due to suppressed desires in the subconscious mind. To free up the subconscious mind Freud developed the technique of hypnotherapy, with which he achieved some great successes. This is because in the hypnotic state, inhibitions are removed and the subconscious mind can express itself; this is very therapeutic.

I often refer patients to a clinical hypnotherapist if they have a lot of psychosomatic symptoms. Hypnotherapy is also effective for quitting bad habits such as smoking.

The father of medicine, Hippocrates was way off track when it came to explaining the cause of the problems women had with their hormones and their sexuality. Hippocrates blamed everything on a wandering uterus! Curiously during history, men's problems have never been explained by a theory of a *wandering penis*!

I remember one evening in the 1980s, relating Hippocrates's theory on the causation of female hormonal and sexual imbalances to an entirely male audience. These men had come to listen to my after-dinner talk about "How to be a perfect husband". My mother had got me into this rather sticky situation, as she had delighted in 'setting me up' when the male dominated Lions Club had requested my services as an after-dinner speaker.

As I explained that Hippocrates had blamed a "wandering uterus that travelled up to the brain and disturbed the emotions", a little man at the front of the audience became wide-eyed and intrigued. I further related that Hippocrates' treatment was to entice the wayward uterus back into its correct position in the pelvis by burning aromatic incense at the vaginal opening. At this juncture, the same man's jaw fell open and he looked relieved. After my light-hearted dissertation, he came up to me and whispered in my ear saying that "he had problems at home and did I have any of that incense for sale!" It is amazing what desperate husbands will do to put their partner in the mood for sex!

The terms *hysteria* or *hysterical illness* were not deleted from psychiatric theories or texts until the 1960s and there were still some text books that I saw in the 1970s that alluded to hysterical illness. Although no longer used, it reminds us that many physical symptoms can be caused by suppressed or frustrated emotions of which we are completely unaware.

The same holds true for suppressed sexuality. If you come from a conservative family background you may have been conditioned during childhood that it's not ladylike or good manners to talk about sexual matters. Even worse if you were a victim of childhood sexual abuse, you may carry very deep and suppressed fears in your subconscious mind; indeed you may be totally unaware of these negative emotions but they could still be causing you anxiety.

Repressed fears and emotions can cause symptoms which include:

• Inability to relax during sex
• Absence of sexual desire
• Pelvic congestion and fullness
• Chronic pelvic pain

- Pain during sexual intercourse
- Spasm of the vaginal muscles (vaginismus)
- Inability to orgasm
- Headaches
- High blood pressure
- Irritable bowel syndrome or irritable bladder
- Skin disorders
- Insomnia
- Anxiety and/or depression

If you suspect these problems may be relevant to you, see your family doctor who can refer you to a good psychologist, a sex therapist and/or a clinical hypnotherapist. Life is too short to put up with these unpleasant symptoms. I often say to patients that chronic stress will make you sicker and kill you quicker than anything.

See resources section in the rear of the publication for more help.

Relevant tests for poor libido

Normal Ranges in the blood

Sex Hormone levels	Men	Women
Total Testosterone	*300-1200 ng/dL*	*30-95 ng/dL*
Free testosterone	*9-30 ng/dL*	*0.3-1.9 ng/dL*
SHBG	*20-60nmol/L*	*40-120nmol/L*

Estrogen levels in a post-menopausal female are less than 130 pmol/L (or less than 35 pg/mL)

Ask your doctor to check your thyroid function because an abnormality in thyroid function can disrupt your sex hormones and reduce libido.

If you are taking hormone therapy check your liver function annually.

Vaginal acid base balance

The acidity of the vaginal mucus membranes and vaginal secretions is important for vaginal health. A healthy vagina is acidic. An unhealthy vagina is alkaline. The healthy vagina is acidic because the lactobacilli living in the vagina make lactic acid.

Acidity is measured as *the pH level* and there are paper strips which measure the pH level that are sold in drug stores. The pH reading on the paper strip should be 3.5 to 4.5 after one minute.

How does your doctor do the vaginal pH test?

The strip of paper is placed against the lower wall of your vagina. Fluid is not tested from the cervix or from the speculum, as the reading will not be accurate. If the test is done on a woman who has had sexual intercourse recently the test will not be accurate as semen is alkaline. If there is any menstrual blood in the vagina the test will not be accurate.

If the vaginal pH is acidic (normal) this indicates the following –

• Friendly lactobacilli are growing and populating the vagina thus keeping away the bad smelly bugs such as trichomonas or streptococci. However yeast such as candida can grow in an acidic vagina.

• Adequate levels of estrogen are being produced in the body

If the vaginal pH is alkaline (too high) = above 4.6 this is not optimal and may indicate –

• Low levels of estrogen

• Bacterial or trichomonal infection in the vagina

• Chronic inflammation in the vagina, which is often also present in the vulva

Conclusion

I wished I had been able to read this book when I was a young woman as it would have given me more self understanding. I grew up in the days before sex was seen on TV and was a subject of education at schools. I remember at the age of 8 years asking my poor mother about sex. I was a curious child and I asked her if one did it standing up or lying down and if it was something you did quickly to get it over with. I also asked her "How often do you do sex?" The voice of my father emanated from the lounge room saying "Not bloody often enough!" Of course at that age I did not get the joke but my father was obviously a typical male. My poor mother was somewhat embarrassed but she did her best to explain it.

It is interesting that when a group of women are relaxing socially together, they will usually talk about their past and present relationships and sex at a much more detailed and open level than they share with men. They often talk about failed or disappointing relationships, which is not surprising as our relationships with our sexual partners teach us a lot about ourselves on many levels. Older women are wiser because of experiences and it is difficult to put an old head on young shoulders. We want our daughters and sons to have good relationships and try to impart our knowledge and wisdom to them.

Hopefully this book has helped you to gain self understanding which can help your relationship with your sexual partner and just as importantly with yourself. Good sex is healthy and fun and can open up a new dimension of enjoyment in your life.

Other titles by Dr Cabot

- *The Liver Cleansing Diet*
- *Fatty Liver - You Can Reverse It*
- *The Breast Cancer Prevention Guide*
- *Diabetes Type 2: A Diet to Reverse it Naturally*
- *Help for Depression and Anxiety*
- *Hepatitis and AIDS - How to fight them naturally*
- *Infertility - The Hidden Causes*
- *Magnesium - The Miracle Mineral*
- *Raw Juices Can Save Your Life*
- *Want to Lose Weight but Hooked on Food?*
- *Can't Lose Weight? - Unlock the Secrets that Keep you Fat*
- *Your Thyroid Problems Solved - Holistic Solutions*
- *Tired of Not Sleeping? Wholistic Program for a Good Night's Sleep*
- *How NOT to kill your husband. Dr Cabot's guide to hormone happiness*

Helpful Resources

World Association for Sexual Health
1300 S. Second Street, Suite 180
Minneapolis, MN 55414
612 625-1500
www.worldsexology.org

Society for the Scientific Study of Sexuality
www.sexscience.org

American Association of Sexuality Educators, Counselors and Therapists
www.aasect.org

American Board of Sexology

American Academy of Clinical Sexologists
www.sexologist.org

American Association for Marriage and Family Therapy
www.aamft.org

American Psychiatric Nurses Association
www.apna.org

American Psychological Association
www.apa.org

American Psychiatric Association
www.psych.org

HERS Foundation – Hysterectomy Educational Resources and Services
www.nafc.org

Society for the Advancement of Women's Health Research
www.hersfoundation.com

The Center for Vulvovaginal Disorders
3 Washington Circle, NW, Suite 205
Washington DC 20037
202 887 0568

National Vulvodynia Association
P. O. Box 4491
Silver Spring MD 20914 - 4491
301 299-0775
www.nva.org

U.S. Vulvar Health Awareness Initiative
P. O. Box 6762
Bloomington, IN 47407
www.vulvarhealth.org

Vulval Pain Society
PO Box 7804
Nottingham
NG3 5ZQ
www.vulvalpainsociety.org

American Physical Therapy Association
1111 N. Fairfax Street
Alexandria VA 22314 - 1488
703 683 6748
www.apta.org

Association for Applied Psychophysiology and Biofeedback
303 422-8436
www.AAPB.org

North American Menopause Society
Mayfield Heights, OH 44124
440 442-7550
www.menopause.org

National Lichen Sclerosis Support Group UK
www.lichensclerosus.org

Compounding Pharmacies

These make bio-identical hormones. Some of them make oxytocin nasal sprays and troches.

USA

Women's International Pharmacy
12012 N. 111th Avenue
Youngtown AZ 85363
800 279-5708
www.womensinternational.com

Australia

Belgian Gardens Pharmacy
47-49 Bundock St,
Belgian Gardens QLD 4810 AUSTRALIA
+61 7 4771 5565

Fresh Theropeutics Broadway
M102 Broadway Healthcare
Level 1 Broadway Shopping Centre
1 Bay Street
Broadway NSW 2007 AUSTRALIA
Phone: +61 2 92 816 816
Fax: +61 2 92 816 862
Email: fresh.broadway@nunet.com.au

West Lindfield Compounding Pharmacy
Graeme Skinner B.Pharm., M.P.S.
30 Moore Avenue, Lindfield, NSW 2070 AUSTRALIA
Phone: + 61 2 9416 2642   Fax: +61 2 9415 6604
order@compoundingchemist.com

References

1. Hormone replacement after cancer, The Lancet. 2004 Feb 7; 363(9407):453-5

2. Biglia N et al, Hormone Replacement Therapy in Cancer Survivors. Maturitas 2004; 48(4):333-346

3. Von Schoultz E. et al, Menopausal Hormone Therapy after Breast Cancer; The Stockholm randomized trial. Journal of the National cancer Institute 2005; 97(7):533-535

4. Batur P. et al, Menopausal Hormone Therapy in Patients with Breast Cancer. Maturitas 2006; 53(2):123-132

Oxytocin

5. Carmichael MS. et al, The Journal of Clinical Endocrinology and Metabolism 64 (1):27-31

6. Carmichael MS. et al, Archives of Sexual Behavior 23 (1):59-79.

7. Marazziti D. et al, Clinical Practice and Epidemiology in Mental Health 2:28, www.ncbi.nlm.nih.gov/pubmed/17034623

Selenium

8. Garlend M. et al, The epidemiology of selenium and human cancer. San Diego, CA; Academic Press; 1994;263-281

Levander OA et al, Selenium and viral virulence, British med Bull 1999; 55(3): 528-533

Selenium Monograph – Alternative Medicine Review. Volume 8, Number 1. 2003

Beck MA et al, Selenium deficiency and viral infection. J Nutr 2003;133 (5 Suppl 1):1463S-7S

Rayman MP. The importance of selenium to human health. Lancet 2000; 356:233-41

Rayman MP, Dietary selenium; time to act, British Medical Journal, Vol. 314, 387, Feb 1997

9. Linda D. Cowan et al. Breast cancer incidence in women with a history of progesterone deficiency. American Journal of Epidemiology Vol. 114, No. 2:209-217.

10. The bio-identical hormone debate, Dr Ken Holtorf, Postgraduate Medicine, Volume 121, Issue 1, January 2009, ISSN - 0032-5481, e-ISSN-1941-9260

11. Tercan M, et al, Facilitated tissue expansion with topical estriol. Department of Plastic and Reconstructive Surgery, Gaziantep University, Turkey.

12. S Koloszár and L Kovács Orv Hetil, Treatment of climacteric urogenital disorders with an estriol-containing ointment, 136 (7):343-5 (1995) PMID 7870416

13. American Journal of Obstetrics & Gynecology. June 1999, 180(6): 1504-11

14. Estrogen Plus Progestin and Breast Cancer Incidence and Mortality in Postmenopausal Women JAMA. 2010;304(15):1684-1692.

15. Significant fall in hormone replacement therapy prescription in general practice Fam Pract. 2010;27(4):424-429.

16. Decision about stopping hormone replacement therapy BMJ. 2010;341(jul07_1):c2421.

17. Rossouw JE, et al. (2002). "Risks and benefits of estrogen plus progestin in healthy postmenopausal women: principal results from the Women's Health Initiative randomized controlled trial". JAMA 288 (3): 321–33.

18. Anderson GL, et al. (2004). "Effects of conjugated equine estrogen in postmenopausal women with hysterectomy: the Women's Health Initiative randomized controlled trial". JAMA 291 (14): 1701–12.